SQUINT

Basic and Clinical Aspects

SQUINT

Basic and Clinical Aspects

J. N. ROHATGI

MS (Pat), MS (Bihar), FRCS (Edin.), FRCS (Eng.),
FRC Opth. (Lond.), FIAMS, FORCE

Formerly
Professor & Head, Department of Ophthalmology, and
Principal, Patna Medical College, and
Ophthalmic Advisor to Government of Bihar, Patna

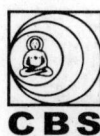

CBS

CBS PUBLISHERS & DISTRIBUTORS
NEW DELHI • BANGALORE

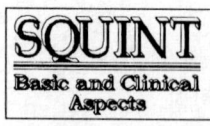

First Edition : 2003

Copyright © 2003, Author and Publishers

ISBN : 81-239-0960-8

Production Director : Vinod K. Jain

Published by :
Satish Kumar Jain for CBS Publishers & Distributors,
4596/1-A, 11 Darya Ganj, New Delhi - 110 002 (India)
E-mail : cbspubs@del3.vsnl.net.in
Website : http://www.cbspd.com

Branch Office :
Seema House, 2975, 17th Cross, K.R. Road,
Bansankari 2nd Stage, Bangalore - 560070
Fax : 080-6771680 • E-mail : cbsbng@vsnl.net

Printed at :
Asia Printograph, Shahdara, Delhi - 110032 (India)

to

my loving grandchildren
Rahul, Rashi, Neha, Ranjan and Nishant

and

my patients
whose beaming smile
after the operation
is my greatest reward

Preface

Strabismus or squint is a fascinating subject. Textbooks of ophthalmology devote exhaustive chapters to ocular motility and its defects. A few textbooks written by eminent eye surgeons dealing with this subject alone are available.

In day-to-day practice, eye surgeons come across cases of squint where parents are anxious for treatment of the cosmetic blemish — least caring for improvement of visual acuity which is reduced in many of these cases. For an eye specialist, diagnostic acumen and relevant treatment of these cases is necessary.

Teachers, consultants and postgraduates in ophthalmology who have deep interest in squint have to know and use the theoretical intricacies, the practical aspects of diagnostic aids and the multifactorial treatment suited to their cases.

The present textbook aims to cater to all categories of ophthalmologists. The language has been kept simple. Obsolete ideas, methods and theoretical conjectures have been excluded. The rationale of various procedures and essential surgical details that would lead to more accurate surgery have been described.

The book may appear to be a one man show but it is not so. In the background have been relevant literature past and present, my teachers, colleagues as also many of my postgraduate students who are now in their own right senior teachers, consultants and successful surgeons. Every chapter of the book has been carefully and exhaustively discussed before being finalised. Though individual opinions have varied, a broad consensual view has prevailed and been described. In the chapter on surgery, buckling or tenoplication (author's nomenclature) has been emphasized as an alternative procedure to resection.

J. N. Rohatgi

Acknowledgement

I have been fascinated about strabismus and its intricacies right from the days when I was a postgraduate student in ophthalmology. I had the pleasure of working under Mr. T. Keith Lyle, an international authority on the subject of squint and the then Dean of the Institute of Ophthalmology and Consultant at Moorfields Eye Hospital, London. I have been greatly benefited by his teaching and monumental book *Practical Orthoptics in the Treatment of Squint*, 1967, published by Henry Kimpton, London, and its subsequent editions.

I have gone through other well known English language books on the subject — Duke Elder's *Textbook of Ophthalmology and System of Ophthalmology, Parson's Textbook of Eye, Von Noorden Binocular Vision and Ocular Motility, Helveston Surgical Management of Strabismus, Peyman's Principles and Practice of Ophthalmology, Modern Ophthalmology* edited by L. C. Dutta 1994 and 1999, etc. as also the various monograms, journals, original articles, comments and discussions on the subject in different seminars, etc. They all have helped in providing me useful thoughts and ideas so necessary in writing a book. At places, I did not hesitate in quoting sentences from them as also incorporating a few of their figures, diagrams and photographs in the present book. I am greatly indebted to these authors and their publishers for this.

This book, though primarily written by me, has been a cooperative effort of a number of senior eye surgeons and teachers in ophthalmology. My colleagues and associates Ajit Sinha, Reyaz Hassan, Bimal Chandra, K. C. Mohanty, B. K. Prasad and N. P. Verma have provided valuable support in many and diverse ways. I am deeply grateful to each one of them. Vijay Bhagat of Bihar Scientific Publication has been a great asset in my efforts.

I owe my sincere thanks to my typists Devendra Prasad and Shri Acharya who have ungrudgingly cooperated in typing and retyping the text at various stages.

CBS Publishers and Distributors' deserve all praise for their valuable suggestions, patience, cooperation and substantially improving the quality of publication.

Most of all, in support of this effort now and from the beginning have been my wife Malti and daughters Anita and Anuja. Their patience and help can never be repaid.

J. N. Rohatgi

Contents

Preface   *vii*

Introduction   *xv*

1. Anatomy of the Extraocular Muscles   1

Rectus Muscles 1
Oblique Muscles 5
The Fascial Structures 6
Tenon's Capsule 7
Muscle Sheaths and their Extensions 8
The Fascial Sheaths of the Recti and Oblique Muscles 9
Blood Supply of the Extraocular Muscles 11
Nerve Supply of the Extraocular Muscles 7
Action of Extraocular Muscles 12
Vertical Muscles 13
Oblique Muscles   13

2. Ocular Movements   15

The Axes of Rotation 15
Versions 16
Primary and Secondary Deviation 21
Vergence 23

3. Binocular Single Vision   26

Retinal Receptors, their Distribution and Corresponding
   Retinal Points 27
Horopter 29
Suppression 32
Kinetic Reflexes Concerned with Accommodation and Convergence 36
Space Perception 37

4. Accommodation–Convergence
State of Convergence and Accommodation
39

Accommodation 39
Convergence 41
Reflex Convergence or Involuntary Convergence 43
Convergence Excess 45
Accommodational Convergence 45

5. Examination and Investigations
51

Preferential Looking 54
Cover-Test 56
Angle of Deviation 59
Fusion 65

6. Sensory Adaptation in Concomitant Squints
Including Amblyopia
67

Diplopia 68
Suppression 69
Abnormal (or Anomalous) Retinal Correspondence 73
Detection of ARC 77
Amblyopia 80
Straight Eye Amblyopia 82
Amblyopia with Squint 84
Fixation Pattern of Amblyopic Eye 85
Pathogenesis of Amblyopia 85
Occlusion 87
CAM Treatment for Amblyopia 90

7. Treatment and Management of Concomitant Strabismus
Medical
94

Divergent Squint Cases 96
Prisms 97
Occlusion 97
CAM Treatment 99
Inverse Occlusion 100
Pleoptic Treatment 100
Treatment with Drugs 103

8. **Surgery for Concomitant Squint**
   Indication and Underlying Principle   **107**

   Infantile Esotropia 108
   Accommodational Convergent Squint 109
   Alternating Convergent Squint 109
   Adjustable Sutures 113
   Faden Operation 115
   Tenoplication (Buckling) 117
   Inferior Oblique Myectomy 122
   Weakening Operation for Superior Oblique 123

9. **Heterophoria**
   Latent Squint   **129**

   Heterophoria 130
   Types of Heterophoria 130
   Extrinsic Ocular Muscle Balance 134
   Cyclophoria 140

10. **Concomitant Squint**
    Heterotropia   **142**

    Concomitant Convergent Strabismus (Esotropia) 142
    Accommodative Esotropia with Convergence Excess
       (or with High Ac/A Ratio) 145
    Partially Accommodative Esotropia (Convergent Strabismus) 145
    Non-Accommodational Convergent Deviation   146
    Essential Infantile Esotropia 146
    Secondary Consecutive Convergent Squint 151

11. **Concomitant–Divergent Strabismus**
    Exotropia   **155**

    Primary Divergent Squint 156
    Secondary Divergent Squint 161
    Consecutive Divergent Squint 162

12. A and V Syndrome
164

13. Vertical Squint
174

Concomitant Vertical Deviations 174
Dissociated Vertical Deviation (DVD) 175
Vertical Deviation and Overaction of the Inferior Oblique
   Muscle (Strabismus Sursoaductorious) 178
Special Group 180

14. Paralytic Squint
182

Examination and Investigation 183
Demonstration of Diplopia 188
Etiology 192

15. Special Forms of Strabismus
Duane's Retraction Syndrome
203

Duane Type I & II
Superior Oblique Tendon Sheath (Brown's) Syndrome 206
Strabismus Fixus 208
Thyroid Myopathy 208
Fracture of the Orbital Floor (Blowout Fracture) 209

16. Nystagmus
211

Etiology and Types 211
Ocular Nystagmus 212
Voluntary Nystagmus 213
Physiologically Induced Ocular Nystagmus 213
Pathological Nystagmus 214
Management of Nystagmus 216

Index
219

Introduction

One of the faculties of the human eye is its ability of binocular single vision, that is to see an object as one despite its images being formed separately on the retinas of the two eyes. And for this function there is an elaborate mechanism — a failure or defect of which produces strabismus or squint resulting sometimes in double vision.

Strabismus or *cross-eye* has been known since the ancient times and its treatment was wrapped in mystery. Legends have it that it is an affliction sent by an angry God and needs or brooks no treatment, notwithstanding the cosmetic embarrassment arising out of such a squinting eye (being well known). The functional defect and poor vision, though no less important, however, get side tracked.

It had been assumed that untreated strabismus would not become worse. That amblyopia and lack of stereopsis (were handicaps) as well as other sensory and motor anomaly would be harder to correct as the child becomes older. Further peripheral fusion with central scotoma, obligatory, persistent, or recurrent amblyopia and abnormal retinal correspondence may be irreparable. Even then early treatment has been hesitatingly done or is not advised even today by a number of ophthalmic medical practitioners.

This malady of squint has been variously mentioned in European medical practice and literature from early 17th Century. Chevalier John Taylor (1703–1721) perhaps realised that squint was a disturbance of muscle-equilibrium and that it could be cured by dividing a muscle, but it has not been known with accuracy whether he carried out tenotomy. In 1829 Anthony White suggested tenotomy as a cure for squint but his attempt was a failure. A little over hundred years thereafter in 1839 Dieffenbach of Berlin performed successfully myotomy of the medial rectus muscle on a seven-year old boy and he could thus be given the priority of introducing surgical measure of treatment.

Strabismus surgery has thereafter, followed a steady course of progress. Improved diagnostic techniques have led to more accurate surgery. Improvement in anaesthesia, sutures and needles after the Second World War and the recent use of botulinum toxin in addition to antibiotics and corticosteroid have broadened the scope of strabismus surgery. Beginning with weakening procedures of the medial rectus, surgery on the oblique muscles is of recent origin because of anatomical difficulty. And now extraocular muscle transfer procedures for a variety of strabismus conditions are being performed.

With these advances more and more ophthalmologists are now emphasising an early correction of the motor anomaly using glasses, miotics, prism and or surgery with the expectation that the sensory mechanism would automatically become normal or nearly normal, specially with the aid of orthoptics.

Statistics could, however, be quoted on both sides, as to whether to treat such children at an early age or as soon as the deviation is obvious, or leave it till the child grows to puberty when it is anticipated that the deviation would go out spontaneously.

It is now becoming increasingly and widely accepted that the latter concept is harmful. Such children, therefore, need urgent attentive treatment and at the earliest possible opportunity.

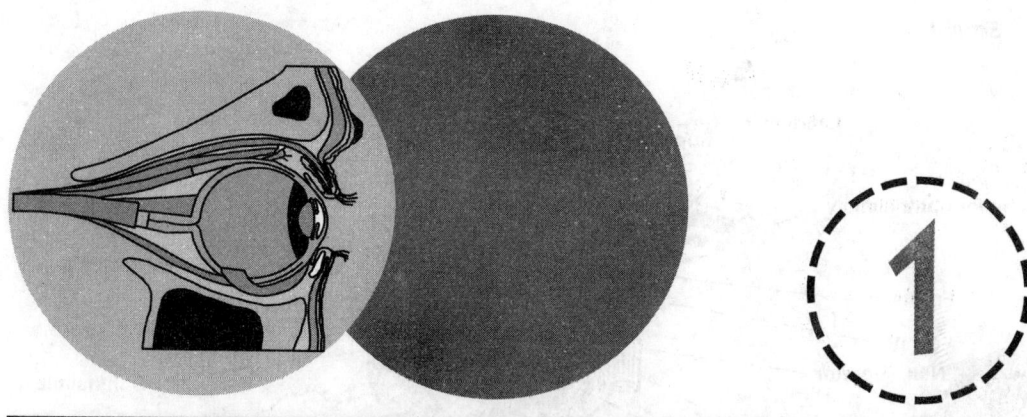

Anatomy of the Extraocular Muscles

There are three pairs of extraocular muscles to each eye, namely, a pair of horizontal recti, the medial and lateral rectus muscles; a pair of vertical recti, the superior and inferior rectus muscles; and a pair of oblique muscles, the superior oblique and the inferior oblique muscles.

A clear knowledge of the anatomy of the extraocular muscles as also of their fascial structures and fat associated with the globe and orbit is a prerequisite to successful strabismus surgery. In addition, their lateral extensions to the lateral and medial orbital wall do play a restrictive role in the extraocular muscle movements.

But before considering these sheaths and fascial attachments, a short descriptive anatomy of the extraocular muscles needs be described.

RECTUS MUSCLES

The rectus muscles are more or less flat, narrow bands that attach themselves with broad thin tendons to the globe.

The origin of these four recti muscles as also of the superior oblique muscle and the levator palpebrae superioris is at the tip of the orbital pyramid (Fig. 1.1). The origin is arranged more or less in a circular fashion, the "annulus of Zinn" surrounding the optic foramen and a part of the superior orbital fissure. Through this opening (surrounded by the origin of these muscles) the optic nerve, the ophthalmic artery and parts of 3rd and 4th cranial nerves enter the muscle cone. The interlocking of muscles and tendon fibres at the origin creates a strong

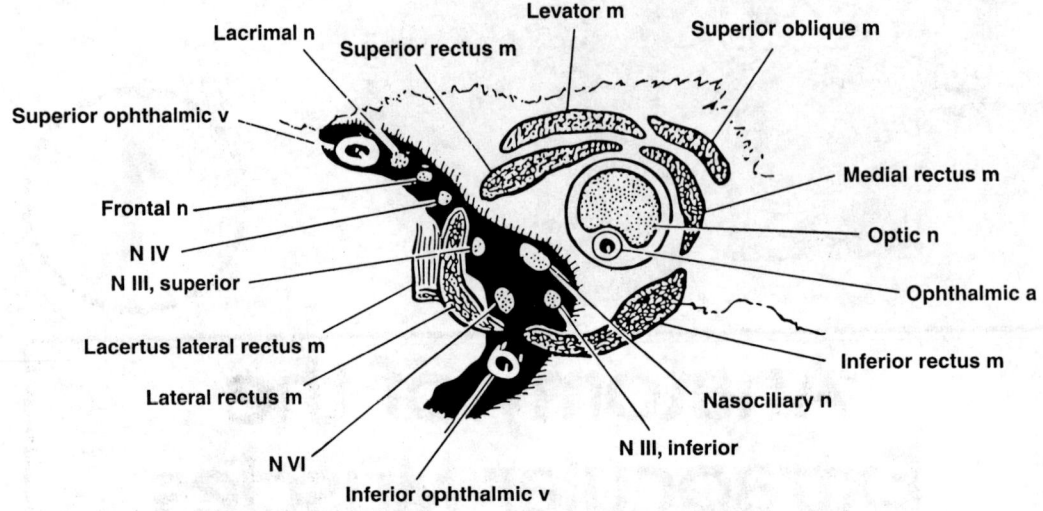

Fig. 1.1: *Topographic relationship of muscle origin around the annulus of Zinn in the posterior part of the orbit.*

anchoring of these extraocular muscles. Attachment exists between the origin of the medial rectus and superior rectus and the dura mater of the underlying optic nerve. This explains the pain occurring on eye movements superiorly and medially in cases of optic neuritis.

Running anteriorly (from the common site of origin) to the eyeball, the medial rectus and lateral rectus muscles follow the corresponding walls of the orbit for a good part of their course. The inferior rectus muscle remains in contact with the orbital floor in the posterior half of the orbit, while the superior rectus muscle is separated from the roof of the orbit by the levator palpebrae superioris muscle (Fig.1.2).

A little in front of the equator, these muscles turn towards the eyeball in a gentle curve and insert on the sclera at varying distances from the limbus. The details of the muscles, their length, length of their tendons and the width of the tendons, etc. are given in Table 1.1.

It is to be noted that in some eyes, recurrent fibres may detach themselves from the bulbar-side of the rectus muscles near their insertion and attach themselves to the sclera, 1 to 5 mm behind the normal insertions. Scobee called these attachments as foot-plates and these have an important role to play in the etiology of esotropia.

Unlike the origin, the insertions or attachments of the four rectus muscles do not form a circle that is concentric with the limbus but rather take the shape of a spiral, called the spiral of Tillaux, as shown in Fig. 1.3. It is so because the muscle insertions are not equidistant from the corneal limbus (Table 1.1). The

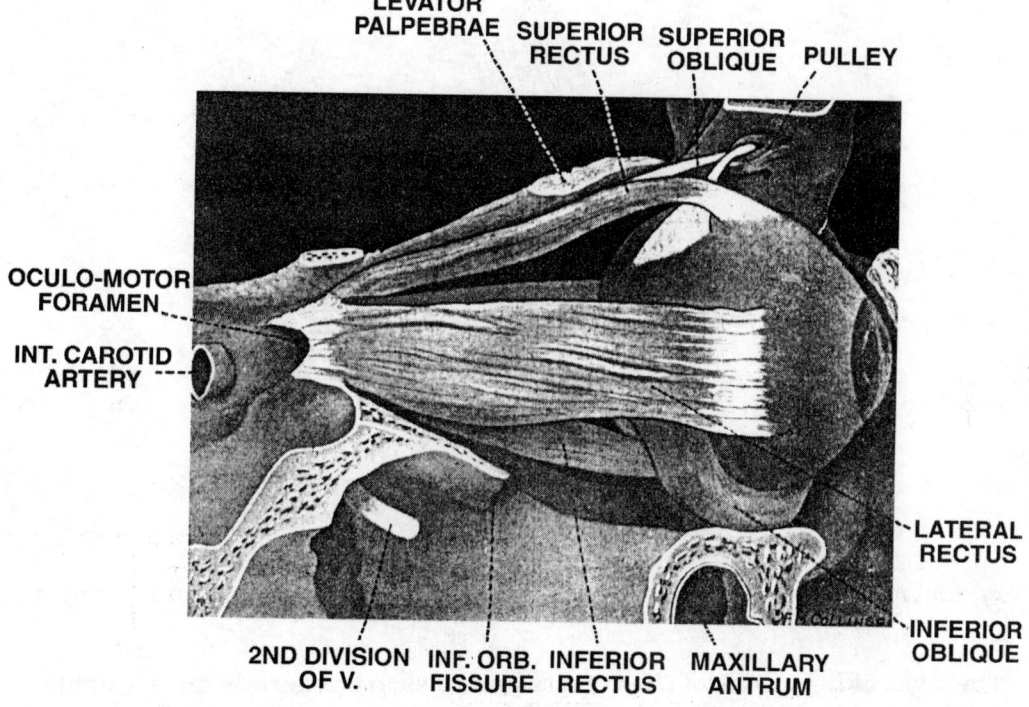

Fig. 1.2: *Ocular muscles in the orbit as seen from the lateral aspect.*

insertion of the medial rectus is closest to the limbus, followed by the inferior, lateral and superior rectus insertions, the superior rectus insertion being the most distant from the corneal limbus.

Table 1.1 Rectus Muscles

(all measurements are in mm)

	Length of muscle	Length of tendon	Width of tendon	Distance of insertion from limbus
1. Medial rectus	37.7 (32.0–44.5)	3.0 (1.0–7.0)	10.4 (8.0–13.0)	5.5 (4.5–7.5)
2. Inferior rectus	37.0 (33.0–42.5)	4.7 (3.0–7.0)	8.6 (7.0–12.0)	6.5 (5.5–8.0)
3. Lateral rectus	36.0 (27.0–42.0)	7.2 (4.0–11.0)	9.6 (8.0–13.0)	6.9 (6.0–9.5)
4. Superior rectus	37.3 (31.0–48.0)	4.3 (2.0–6.0)	10.4 (7.0–12.0)	7.7 (6.5–10.0)

From Lang et al: *Binocular Vision and Ocular Motility*, 4th edn, Noorden, 1990.[5]

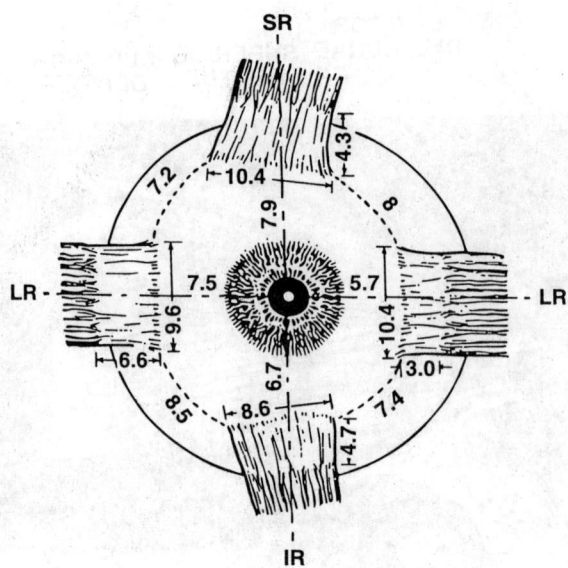

Fig. 1.3: *Insertion of rectus muscles on the scleral surface — distance in mm from limbus.*

The lines of insertions of these rectus muscles are generally not straight. In case of medial and lateral rectus muscles, the linear insertion is often slightly convex towards the corneal limbus. In case of superior rectus and inferior rectus muscles, the lines of insertions are markedly convex towards the corneal limbus and run obliquely upwards and laterally. This results in temporal ends of their insertion being more distant from the corneal limbus than their nasal ends.

Table 1.2 gives important data when it comes to surgery for esotropia or exotropia in children below the age of three years.

It shows a substantial difference of mean anatomical data obtained from adult and new born eyes. Thus, whereas the distance of the middle of insertion of a

Table 1.2 **Medial and Lateral Rectus Muscles in Adults and New Born* (in mm)**

Length of muscle	Width of muscle	Distance from limbus (middle of insertion)
Medial rectus 37.7 (28)	10.4 (7.9)	5.7 (3.9)
Lateral rectus 36.3 (31.6)	9.6 (6.9)	7.5 (4.8)

From Lang et al, quoted from Von Noorden[5]: *Binocular Vision and Ocular Motility*, 4th edn, 1990.
*Figures in parentheses indicate the measurement for new born.

medial rectus muscle from the limbus is taken as an average of 5.7 mm, it is sometimes 3.9 mm in the new born. Similarly it is 4.8 mm for lateral rectus in a new born as against an average of 7.5 mm in an adult eye.

OBLIQUE MUSCLES

Originating from above and medial to the optic foramen, the superior oblique muscle runs along the upper part of the medial wall of the orbit anteriorly to reach the trochlea. The trochlea is a tube 4 to 6 mm long formed medially by a groove, the trochlear fossa" in the frontal bone. Laterally, above and below the wall of the trochlear tube is composed of connective tissues that may contain cartilaginous or bony elements. After passing through this trochlear tube, the superior oblique muscle turns posterolaterally forming an angle of 54° with the pretrochlear or direct portion of the muscle. The muscle becomes tendinous even before entering the trochlear tube (distal third of the direct portion) and continues as a tendon through the trochlear pully and, thereafter, in its entire reflected or post-trochlear part. The tendon passes laterally, backwards and downwards under the superior rectus muscle. It fans out and gets attached to the sclera in the postero-temporal quadrant forming a concave curved line. The width of the insertion varies greatly but is 11 mm on an average. The anterior end of the insertion lies 3 to 4.5 mm behind the lateral end of the insertion of the superior rectus muscle (Fig. 1.4).

The posterior end of the insertion lies 13.6 mm behind the medial end of the insertion of the superior rectus muscle.

Surrounding the muscle tendon in the trochlear tube is a fibrillar vascular sheath. A bursa-like structure is also described between the trochlear saddle

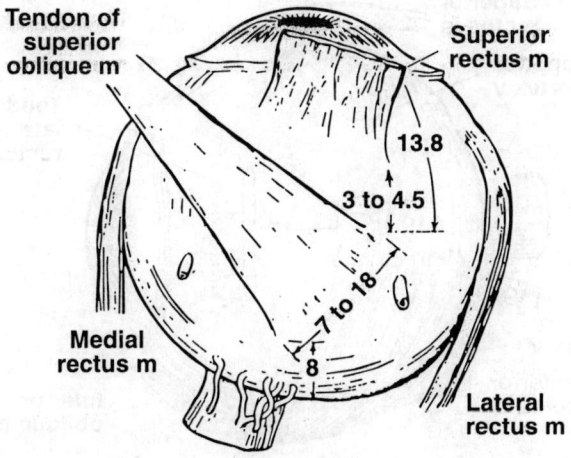

Fig. 1.4: *Insertion of superior oblique tendon and its relationship to superior rectus measurement (in mm) of the insertion.*

and the vascular sheath which may get fibrosed and restrict the movement of superior oblique muscle (Brown's superior oblique sheath syndrome).

Inferior Oblique Muscle

It is the shortest of the extraocular muscles, being 37 mm long. It is almost wholly muscular unlike the other extraocular muscles. Arising in the antero inferior angle of the bony orbit, in a shallow depression in the orbital plate of the maxilla near the lateral edge of the lacrimal fossa, the muscle runs backwards, laterally and upwards passing between the floor of the orbit and the inferior rectus muscle.

The insertion is in the inferotemporal portion of the sclera in the lower half of the eye behind the equator by a short tendon (1 to 2 mm). The width of the insertion tendon varies—on an average it is about 9 mm. The insertion forms a curved concave line; its anterior margin is about 10 mm to 12 mm behind the lower edge of the insertion of the lateral rectus muscle and the posterior end is 2 mm below and 1 to 2 mm lateral to the macula (Fig. 1.5).

The inferior oblique muscle forms an angle of 51° with the vertical plane of the eyeball. It is also unique in its anatomical relationship. It behaves as though it has two potential insertions and two potential points of origin. As the muscle is innervated near its middle, it may be weakened (the most common operation on this muscle) either proximal or distal to its point of innervation.

THE FASCIAL STRUCTURES

The fascial structures in relation to extraocular muscle are tenon's capsule, the muscle-sheaths and their extensions, the check ligaments and the ligament of

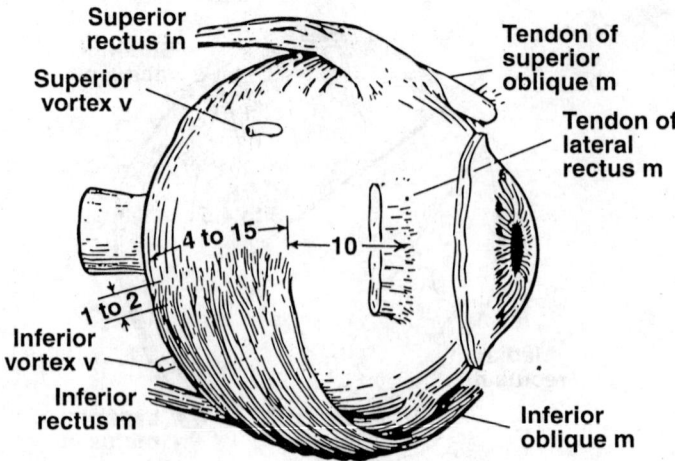

Fig. 1.5: *Inferior oblique muscle — course and relationship of its tendon (measurement in mm of the insertion).*

lockwood, etc. Before describing them, a few lines about the overall covering of the eyeball (in its anterior part), viz. the conjunctiva needs description.

The bulbar-conjunctiva is fused to the underlying anterior tenon's capsule rather loosely except at the limbus. It covers the anterior part of the eyeball from the fornices above (superior) to the fornix below (the inferior fornix) and laterally from the medial to the lateral canthus. It is highly vascular and has a number of small embedded arterioles and veins (branches of the anterior ciliary arteries and of marginal arcades of the lids). These have to be taken care of while incising the conjunctiva to approach underlying tenon's capsule and muscle to avoid undue bleeding at operation for strabismus.

In children the conjunctiva and its attached underlying tenon's capsule is thick but becomes thinner, fibrillar and friable in adults and old age.

In the inferior fornix, lying underneath the conjunctiva is a pad of fat which is about 12 to 14 mm from the limbus (its anterior extension) and, therefore, it is necessary that while incising the conjunctiva in the inferior fornix to expose the sclera, the line of incision should be anterior to this pad of fat not more than 12 mm behind or from the limbus. This also avoids injury to the line of attachment of posterior tenon's capsule.

An incision carried too deeply in the fornix causes unnecessary bleeding. And a transconjunctival incision should not be made over the insertion of the medial or lateral rectus muscles but a few millimeters behind the line of insertion, otherwise it would produce an unsightly scar which may also sometimes restrict the ocular motility.

In the medial part of the interpalpebral opening is a fold of conjunctiva, the plica senilunaris and just medial to it is the caruncle. While cutting or repairing conjunctival incision care should be taken to avoid distorting their position otherwise it may lead to cosmetic embarrassment.

Tenon's Capsule

This capsule is a condensation of fibrous tissue that covers the eyeball from the entrance of the optic nerve behind to the limbus anteriorly where it gets firmly fused to the overlying conjunctiva. Except for these areas of fusion, the two structures are separated by the subconjunctival space. Tenon's capsule is also separated from the underlying sclera and in between lies the episcleral space (Tenon's space).

It is divided into an anterior and a posterior part. The anterior portion of the tenon's capsule overlies the anterior half to two-thirds of the rectus muscle as well as the intermuscular space and membrane and is fused loosely to the underlying surface of the bulbar conjunctive being attached to the sclera at limbus.

The posterior portion of the tenon's capsule is composed of the fibrous sheath of the rectus muscles together with the intermuscular membrane. Anteriorly the fibrous attachments between the inner surface of anterior tenon's capsule and the outer muscle sheath (which is in fact posterior tenon's capsule) fuse together at a point 15 to 20 mm behind the insertion of the medial and lateral rectus muscles to form a barrier to extraconal-orbital fat. The lateral attachments between the outer surface of the anterior tenon's capsule and the orbital rim medially and laterally are called check ligaments.

The posterior tenon's capsule is made up of the muscle sheaths or capsule and the intermuscular membrane in between them. This forms a rather capsular bag around the globe (posterior half). The extent to which this intermuscular membrane has been dissected determines how far the muscle specially the medial and lateral recti would retract during surgery.

Orbital fat is present outside anterior tenon's capsule anteriorly and outside posttenon's capsule posteriorly. The tenon's capsule is pierced posteriorly by the optic nerve and around this by ciliary nerves and arteries, just behind the equator by vena-vorticose and anteriorly by the six extrinsic muscles of the eye (Fig. 1.6).

Muscle Sheaths and their Extensions

The external ocular muscles pierce the tenon's capsule, enter the sub-capsular space and insert into the sclera. And thus one can define an extracapsular and an intracapsular portion of each muscle.

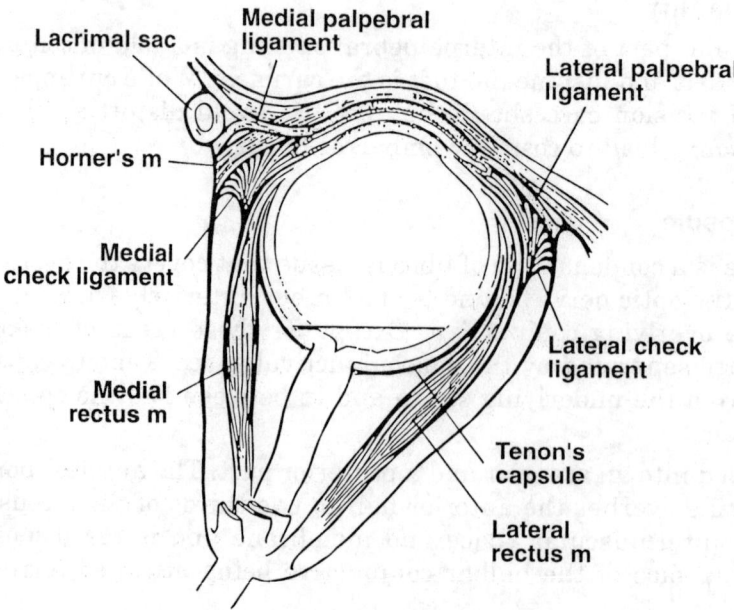

Fig. 1.6: *Tenon's capsule — its reduplication forming muscle-sheath of rectus muscles.*

Each of these muscles in its extracapsular part or posteriorly has a covering called muscle sheath, which is actually the posterior tenon's capsule. This sheath covers the muscle running backwards for a distance of 10 to 12 mm. The muscle sheaths of the four rectus muscles are connected by an intermuscular membrane which is a fascial condensation joining the lateral/medial margins of the four rectus muscle sheaths (Fig. 1.7). In addition numerous fascial extensions pass amongst these sheath making an intricate system of fibrous attachments, with extensions attaching them to the orbit and supporting the eyeball, and thereby controlling the ocular movements from going astray.

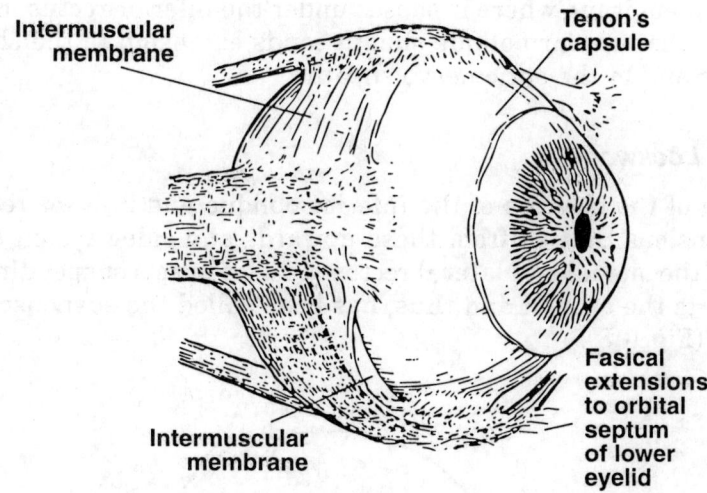

Fig. 1.7: *Intermuscular membrane between the rectus muscles.*

The Fascial Sheaths of the Recti and Oblique Muscles

The medial and lateral recti possess well developed and well-defined fibrous membranes that extend laterally from the muscle sheaths to the respective walls of the orbit and are known as check-ligaments. In case of medial rectus the attachment is to the lachrymal bone behind the posterior lachrymal crest and to the orbital septum behind. In case of lateral rectus, the attachment is to the orbital tubercle on the mallor bone.

The expansion of the fasical sheaths from the superior rectus is attached to the levator palpebrae superiosis by a definite band in which a bursa has been defined by Motais. The band ensures the synergic action of the two muscles—the superior rectus and levator palpebrae superioris. And so when the eye looks upwards (contraction of the superior rectus), the upper lid is raised as well. The fascial sheath of the inferior rectus divides anteriorly into two layers, an upper one which becomes part of the tenon's capsule and a lower one which is about

12 mm long and ends in the fibrous tissue between the tarsus of the lower lid and the orbicularis muscle. This lower portion forms part of the Lockwood's ligament. By this attachment, the inferior rectus can act on the lower lid as the levator acts on the upper lid.

The fascial sheath of the superior oblique covers the reflected part of the muscle and its tendon. Attachments pass from this sheath to the sheath of the levator palpebrae superioris, to the superior rectus sheath and to the tenon's capsule behind above and laterally.

The fascial sheath of the inferior oblique muscle covers the entire muscle. Thin at the origin, it thickens as the muscle runs laterally and develops into a rather dense membrane where it passes under the inferior rectus muscle. Near the insertion, the inferior oblique sheath sends extension to the sheath of the lateral rectus and to the optic nerve sheath.

Ligament of Lockwood

The blending of the sheaths of the inferior oblique and inferior rectus muscle and the extensions that go from these upwards and sideways on each side to the sheath of the medial and lateral rectus muscles form a suspending hammock which supports the eyeball and thus, has been called the suspensory ligament of Lockwood (Fig. 1.8).

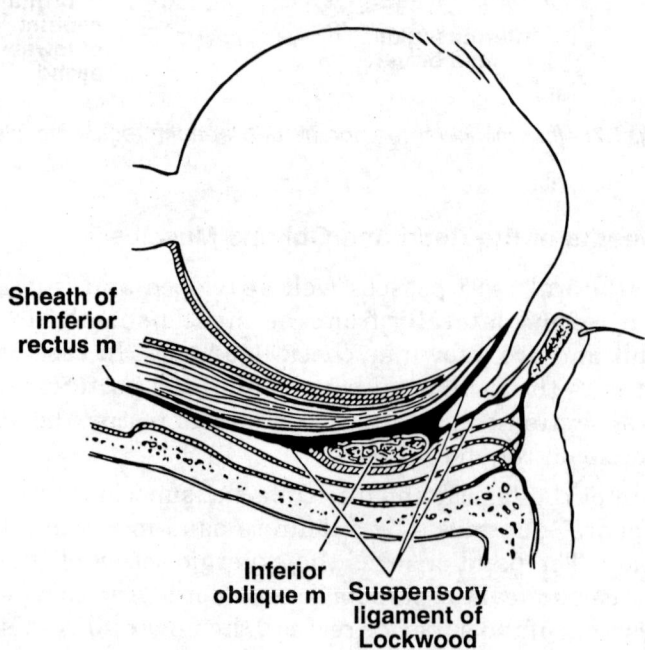

Fig. 1.8: *Suspensory ligament of Lockwood.*

Blood Supply of the Extraocular Muscles

The lateral and superior rectus muscles get their blood supply from the lateral muscular branch of the ophthalmic artery. The superior oblique muscle as also the levator palpebare superioris muscle get their supply from the same lateral muscular branch.

The medial muscular branch of the ophthalmic artery (which is larger than the lateral muscular branch) supplies the medial rectus, inferior rectus, and the inferior oblique muscle. In addition, the medial rectus muscle receives a branch from the lacrymal artery. The inferior oblique and inferior rectus also receive a branch from the infraorbital artery.

From these muscular branches arise the anterior ciliary arteries. Two anterior ciliary arteries emerge from each muscle except for the lateral rectus muscle which has only one. But variations in this number are not uncommon. These anterior ciliary arteries give branches for vascular supply to episclera, sclera, bulbar conjunctiva and limbal area. They pierce the sclera a few mm behind the limbus, cross the underlying superior choroidal space to terminate in the anterior part of the ciliary body. Here they anastomose with the lateral and medial long ciliary arteries to form the major arterial circle of the iris. Hence, damage to the anterior ciliary arteries in squint surgery may cause anterior segment ischaemia. The venous drainage from the extraocular muscle corresponds to the arterial branches and empties into the superior and inferior orbital veins respectively.

Nerve Supply of the Extraocular Muscles

The superior rectus muscle gets its nerve supply from the upper division of the third or oculomotor nerve. The various branches of nerve enter the muscle at the junction of its middle and posterior third. The inferior division of the third nerve supplies the medial rectus, the inferior rectus and the inferior oblique. The branches for the medial rectus muscle enter its belly 15 mm from the origin of the muscle. The branches for the inferior rectus enter the muscle belly at the junction of its posterior and middle thirds. The branches for the inferior oblique enter the muscle just after the muscles passes lateral to the inferior rectus muscle. The lateral rectus has its own independent nerve supply from the 6th or abducent nerve, branches of which enter the muscle 15 mm from its origin on the bulbar side.

The superior oblique muscle is supplied by branches from the 4th or trochlear nerve. Three or four branches of the nerve enter the muscle from the orbital surface. The most anterior enters the muscle belly at the junction of the posterior and middle third of the muscle and the most posterior branch enters the muscle at about 8 mm from its origin.

Action of Extraocular Muscles

To determine whether the patient has a paretic or a concomitant deviation or squint, the examiner must be able to evaluate the action of the extraocular muscles. Such movements are uniocular as also conjugate.

Uniocular movements are called duction, adduction and obduction, while the synchronous and simultaneous movement of the extraocular muscles of the two eyes together is called version, viz. dextroversion, laevoversion, etc.

The action of the medial and lateral rectus muscles are the least complex thus, while medial rectus has the sole function of adduction or medial rotation of the eyeball, the lateral rectus carries out abduction or lateral rotation of the eye (Table 1.3).

Table 1.3 Actions of Extrinsic Ocular Muscles

Muscle	Main action primary	Subsidiary action	
		Secondary	Tertiary
Medial rectus	Adduction		
Lateral rectus	Abduction		
Superior rectus	Elevation	Intorsion	Adduction
Inferior rectus	Depression	Extorsion	Adduction
Superior oblique	Intorsion	Deprassion	Abduction
Inferior oblique	Extorsion	Elevation	Abduction

The vertically acting muscle-superior and inferior recti as also the superior and inferior oblique muscles have complex actions because the axes of the muscles (mainly the obliques) are not parallel with the axis of the eyeball.

Thus, the superior rectus is an elevator, adductor and an intortor. The interior rectus is a depressor, extorter and an adductor. The superior oblique muscle is an intortor (causes the 12 O'clock position of cornea to rotate towards the nose) a depressor and abductor of the eye while the inferior oblique muscle is an extortor (causing temporal rotation of 12 O'clock position of cornea) an elevator and an abductor.

Thus, when vertically acting muscles are considered, their actions are primary, secondary and tertiary.

For superior rectus, the primary action is elevation, that of inferior rectus depression, the superior oblique intorsion and that of inferior oblique extorsion or excyclodeviation.

VERTICAL MUSCLES

The planes of the superior and inferior rectus muscles are assumed to concide at least for clinical purposes. This common muscle plane in primary position forms an angle of about 25° with the antero-posterior axes of the eyeball. Thus when the eye is abducted about 25°, the axis of the superior rectus muscle becomes parallel to the axis of the eyeball and then the superior rectus becomes a pure elevator. In this position of the eye, the inferior rectus is simply a depressor of the eye and its action no longer has an incycloducting component. Because of this inclination, the superior rectus in the primary position of the eye takes it up (elevator) adducts it and also rotates it round the antero-posterior axis causing incycloducttion (inward rotation of the 12 O'clock position of the cornea). The greater the globe is adducted the greater is the incycloduction effect.

In the primary position, the inferior rectus depresses the globe because it is attached to the globe from below. There is also a slight adducting action. Again because of the 25° inclination of the inferior rectus to the antero-posterior axis of the eyeball, when the globe is abducted to this extent) the inferior rectus is not only a pure depressor of the globe, but also causes excyloduction. And thus, in this abducted position of the globe, the incycloduction caused by superior rectus gets neutralised by the excycloduction produced by the inferior rectus.

OBLIQUE MUSCLES

The muscle plane of both superior and inferior oblique muscles go in a direction from the anteromedial aspect to the posterolateral aspect (the area of insertion). Thus neither muscle plane concides with the median plane of the eyeball, nor does the axis of rotation concide with the horizontal axis of the eyeball. As a result of these, in the primary straight ahead position of the globe, the superior oblique causes in-turning (incycloduction) and depression of the globe and also acts as an abductor. When the globe is adducted (action of the medial rectus), the angle between the median plane (anterior-posterior axis of the eyeball) and the muscle plane is reduced completely. The superior oblique becomes more and more depressor. On the other hand when the globe is abducted (lateral rectus action), this angle increases and the superior oblique causes more of incycloduction. For the inferior oblique, similar considerations apply. In primary position it causes excyloduction, elevation and abduction of the globe. When the eye is adducted fully, it causes maximum elevation and when the eye is abducted fully, it produces excycloduction to the utmost extent.

Quite often, along with a third cranial nerve palsy, the patient also has a fourth nerve palsy. In such a situation, it becomes a herculean task to decide whether the 4th cranial nerve is also paralysed. We cannot evaluate the patient's ability to depress the adducted eye. Because of the medial rectus palsy, there is more or less no adduction of the eyeball. Hence the only course is to evaluate the intorting action of the superior oblique (maximum in abduction position). Ask the patient to look down and in position and observe one of the blood vessels adjacent to the cornea to see if it is rotating. If it does intort, or shows rotation towards the nose, its action is present. The superior oblique is therefore not paretic.

REFERENCES

1. Duke Elder, S. and Wybar K. C.: The anatomy of the visual system, *System of Ophthalmology*, Vol. 2, St. Louis, The C. V. Mosby Co, 1961.
2. Fink, W. H.: *Surgery of the Vertical Muscles of the Eye*, 2nd edn, Springfield, Ill., Charles C. Thomas, 1962.
3. Scobee, R. C.: Anatomical factors in the etiology of strabismus. *Am. J. Ophthalmol.*, 31: 781, 1948.
4. Wolff, E.: *Anatomy of the Eye and Orbit*, 6th edn, revised by Last, R. J. Philadelphia, H. K. Lewis & Co. Ltd., 1968.
5. Noorden, G. K. von: *Binocular Vision and Ocular Motility*, 4th edn, C. V. Mosby Co, 1990.

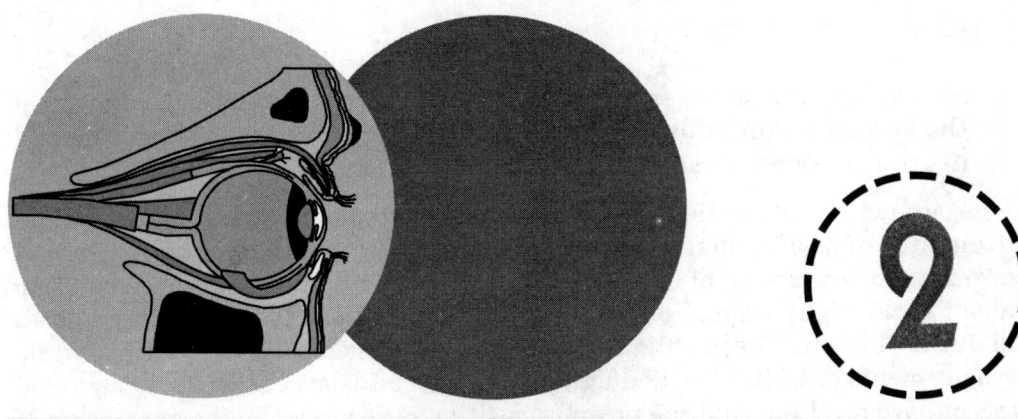

Ocular Movements

The eye (eyeball) rotates around one of the three axes and all of them pass through the centre of rotation. This point or centre of rotation (in primary position) is localised about 13.5 mm (in myopes 14.5 mm) behind the apex of the cornea on the visual axis (the line of sight) and this is 1.35 mm behind the equatorial plane.

THE AXES OF ROTATION

The three axes are explained in Fig. 2.1.

1. *Antero-posterior or sagital axis* (Y-axis in the sketch) which corresponds to the line of vision or fixation, Rotation of the eyeball around this axis leads to intorsion or extorsion that is, tilting of the 12 O'clock position of the cornea (or the upper pole of the cornea) nasally or temporally respectively.

2. *Vertical axis* (Z-axis in the sketch) rotation around which produces adduction (nasal-ward movement) and abduction movement to the temporal side).

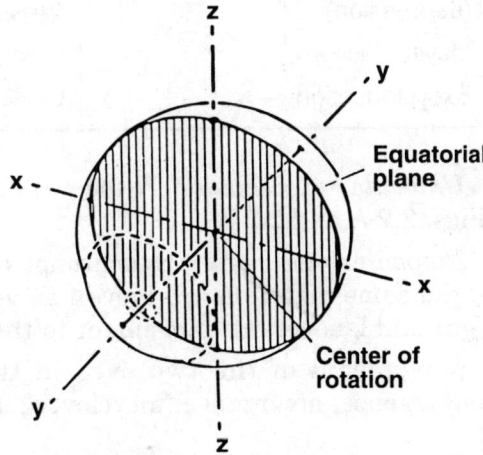

Fig. 2.1: *The three axes of eye: xx horizontal axis, yy antero-posterior axis, zz vertical axis.*

3. *Horizontal axis* or the transverse axis X (from right to left). A rotation of the eyeball around this axis produces vertical movement of elevation and depression deorsumduction).

The adduction, abduction, elevation and depression are the four cardinal movements of the eyeball. A combination of the horizontal and vertical movements or excursion of the globe takes the eye into oblique positions of up and out to the right, up and out to the left, down and out to the right and down and out to the left. These oblique positions are termed tertiary position while the movements of adduction, abduction, elevation and depression are designated as secondary position. And the primary position is assumed by the eyeball when one is looking straight ahead with the body and head erect (see Table 2.1).

A simple terminology for the ocular movement, uniocular and binocular, is as follows (as suggested by Lancaster[8] and quoted by Von-Noorden[10] in *Binocular Vision and Ocular Motility,* 4th edn, 1990).

Table 2.1 Monocular and Binocular Movements of the Eyeball

Monocular movements Duction	Binocular movements	
	Version	Vergence
Adduction	Extroversion	Convergence
Abduction	Laevoversion	Divergence
Sursumduction (elevation)	Sursumversion (elevation)	Right sursumvergence (left deosumvergence)
Deorsumduction (depression)	Deorsumversion (depression)	Right deosumvergence (left sursumvergence)
Incycloduction	Dextrocycloversion	Incyclovergence
Excycloduction	Laevocycloversion	Excyclovergence

Uniocular movements: These are ductions as abduction and adduction, etc. (Figs. 2.2 A and 2.2 B).

Binocular movements: Synchronous simultaneous movements of the two eyes in the same direction are known as versions—dextroversion movement to the right and laeoversion movement to the left (Figs 2.3 A, 2.3 B and 2.3 C).

Movements of the two eyes in the opposite directions are vergence—convergence, divergence, incyclovergence and excylovergence, etc.

VERSIONS

These synochronous and simultaneous movements may be to the right dextroversion, or to the left laeoversion, sursumversion (elevation),

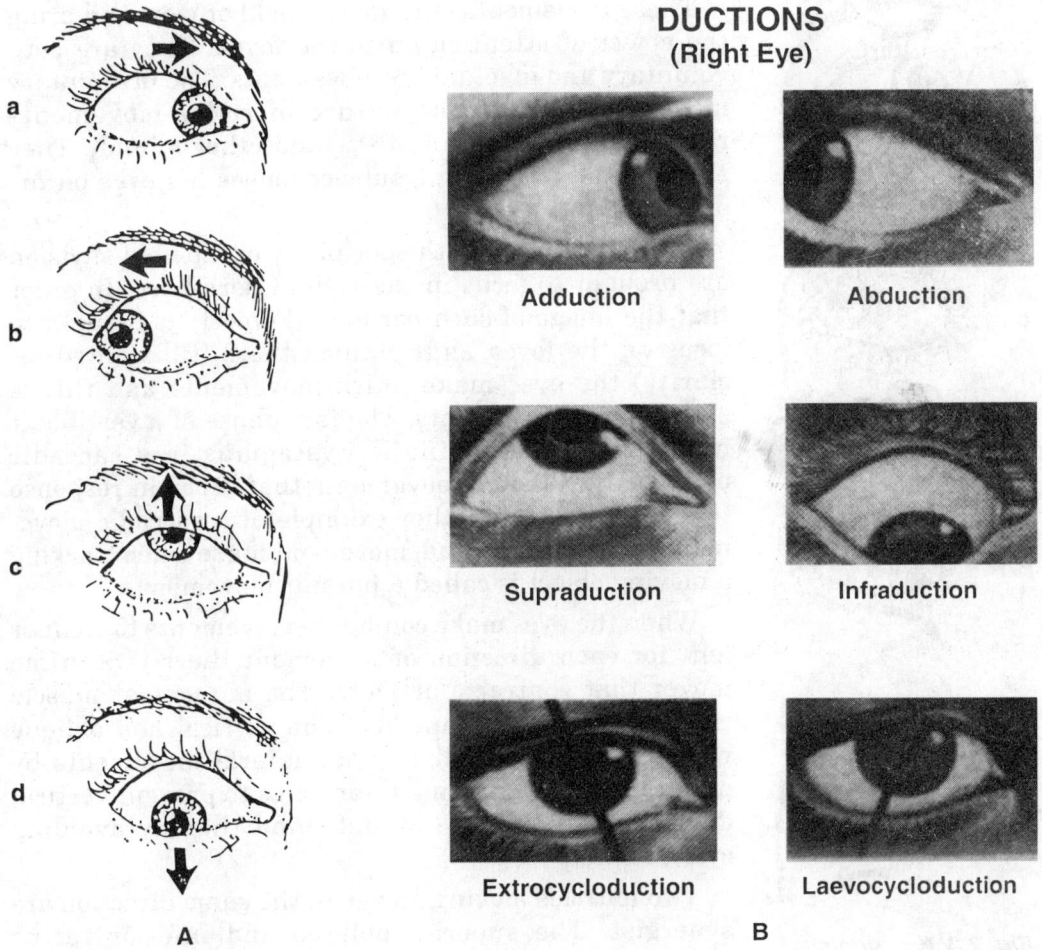

DUCTIONS
(Right Eye)

Adduction	Abduction
Supraduction	Infraduction
Extrocycloduction	Laevocycloduction

A   **B**

Fig. 2.2: **A** *Uniocular movements of eyeball; right eye (duction) secondary positions.* **a.** *Adduction,* **b.** *abduction,* **c.** *elevation (sursumduction),* **d.** *depression (deorsumduction).*
B *Photographic representation right eye ductions.*

deorsumduction (depression) up and out to the right (dextrocycloversion) up and out to the left (laevocycloversion) down and out to the right and down and out to the left.

Table 2.2 shows the muscles mainly concerned in the nine cardinal positions for conjugate movements.

These are extraordinary fast movements. The eyes accelerate sharply early in the movement, reach a maximum velocity and then decelerate gradually. The measurement is in angular velocity and the range is as wide as 30° to 700° per second with a latency of 200 msec. The movements are performed in a such a manner as to minimize an overshoot.

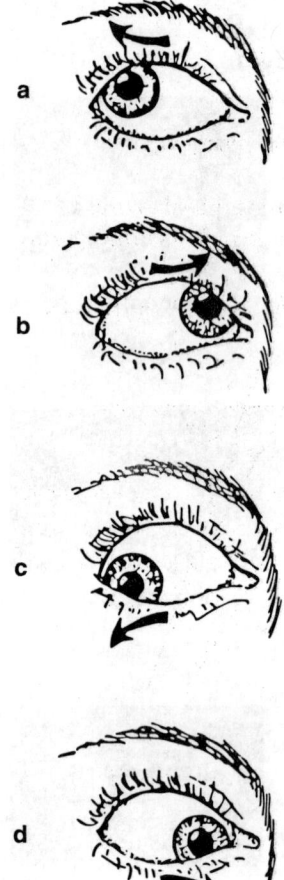

Fig. 2.3 A: *Binocular movements: Some tertiary positions of right eye.* **a.** *Dextroelevation,* **b.** *laevoelevation,* **c.** *dextrodepression, d. laevodepression.*

These movements enlarge the field of view and bring the object of attention on to the fovea. They are both voluntary and involuntary movements. The involuntary movements are of the nature of reflex-movements responding to ocular, acoustic and other stimuli. They are voluntary when the subject moves his eyes on his own volition.

Objects situated in the periphery of the field of vision are brought to focus in the retinal periphery. In order that the image of such peripheral objects is brought to focus on the fovea and retained there (till wanted for clarity) the eyes make quick movements and this is saccadic eye movements. The fast phase of a vestibular nystagmus or optokinetic nystagmus is a saccadic movement. Random movements that occur in response to a command is another example of a saccadic movement. On the other hand, movement made when tracking a moving object is called a pursuit movement.

When the eyes make conjugate movements to right or left, for each direction of movement there is a prime mover that contracts actively. The antagonist muscle receives inhibitory impulses. The vertical and oblique muscles help in stabilising the lateral movements by maintaining or adjusting their tones to prevent vertical deviations of the line of sight and thereby avoiding cyclorotation.

Two muscles moving an eye in the same direction are synergist. The superior oblique and inferior rectus muscles are both depressors of the eye and are as such synergists. When a muscle moves the eye in a direction opposite to the prime mover (agonist), it is an antagonist. Thus, with the movement inwards of an eye by medial rectus, the medial rectus is an agonist, and with movement of the eye laterally, the lateral rectus is agonist.

The two medial and lateral recti are, however, antagonist because the two move the eye in opposite directions. Similar considerations apply to the oblique version movements. The muscles less engaged in performing the vertical rotations stabilise the line of sight. The horizontal muscles bring the eyes to the required lateral or median position. They also assist in extreme positions of elevation and depression.

The divergence of the two visual lines in elevation and distance fixation, as also their relative convergence when looking down and in near-fixation, is

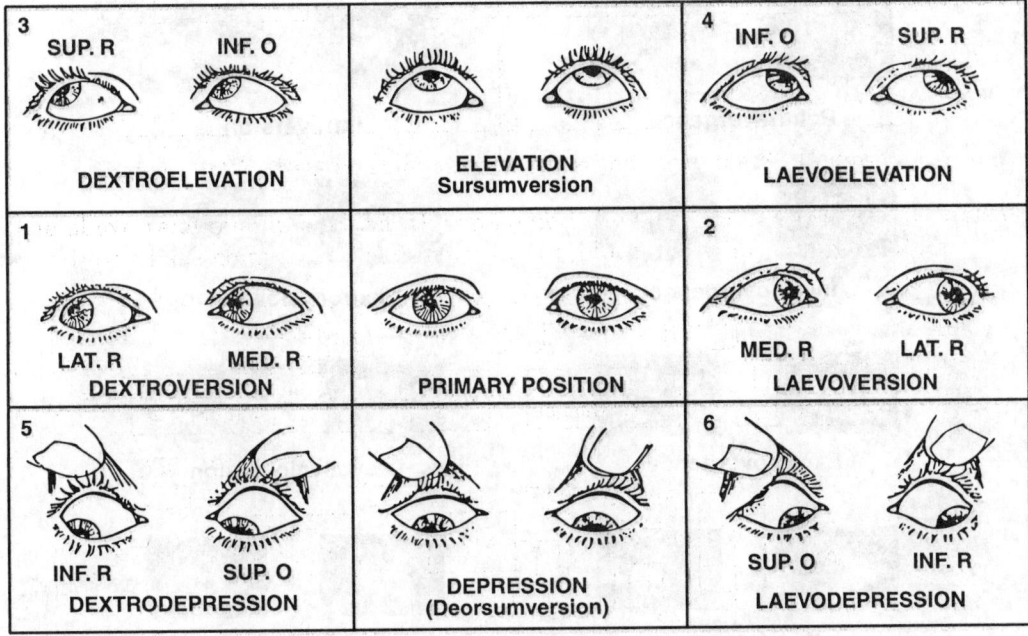

Fig. 2.3 B: *Binocular movements.*

Table 2.2 Muscles of the Eye Concerned with the Nine Cardinal Positions for Conjugate Movements

Dextro elevation	Elevation	Laevo elevation
Right superior rectus	Right superior rectus, Left superior rectus	Right inferior oblique
Left inferior oblique	Right inferior oblique Left inferior oblique	Left superior rectus
Dextro version	Primary Position	Laevo version
Right lateral rectus		Right medial rectus
Left medial rectus		Left lateral rectus
Dextro depression	Depression	Laevo depression
Right inferior rectus	Right inferior rectus Left inferior rectus	Right superior oblique
Left superior oblique	Right superior oblique Left superior oblique	Left inferior rectus

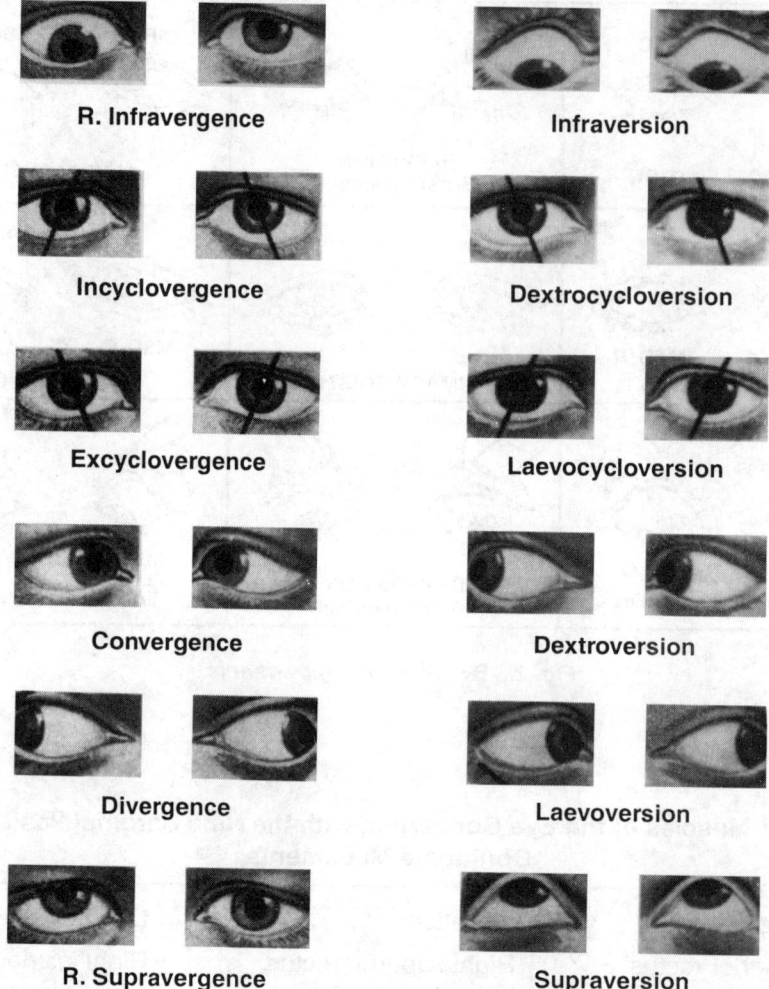

R. Infravergence

Infraversion

Incyclovergence

Dextrocycloversion

Excyclovergence

Laevocycloversion

Convergence

Dextroversion

Divergence

Laevoversion

R. Supravergence

Supraversion

Fig. 2.3 C: *Photographs of binocular movements. Left side vergence movement, right side version movement.*

interpreted as a learned association since there is no change in accommodation for a given convergence position when the eyes are elevated or depressed. Herring, on the contrary, explained it as a result solely of mechanical factors in the relationship of the elevator and depressor muscles.

As regards normal occurring movements of cycloversion, they are considered as postural reflexes. They arise from stimuli in neck muscles and the internal ear. With every change in the position of the head or body, the endolymph in the semicircular canal (of the inner ear) is stimulated. This causes a change of tonus of the extraocular muscle. The changes in the relative tonus within the eye muscles are such that each labyrinth tends to pull each eye towards its side but since the effect of the two labyrinths is equal and antagonist, no change in the position of the eyes takes place when the head is erect and straight.

With every change of the position of the head and body, a change in tonic tension of the extraocular muscles occurs that prevents the eyes from following the rotation of the head. This allows a rotation of the eyes to the left when the head is turned to the right and a rotation of the eyes to the right when the head is turned to the left. When the head is lifted up, the eyes go down and when the head is lowered the eyes go up.

On tilting of the head to one shoulder, say tilting off the head to the right shoulder, the right superior rectus and right oblique muscle (mainly inferior oblique) and the left inferior rectus and oblique (mainly the superior oblique) cooperate in producing a laevoversion of the eye. In other words the upper muscles of the eye on the side towards which the head is tilted and lower muscles of the opposite eye receive active impulses to contract with relaxation of the corresponding antagonist. This is a static reflex originating from the otoliths in the inner ear. Human eyes compensate only to a small extent for the tilting of the head to one shoulder. A quick tilting of the head may result in a cyclorotation of as much as 20° but this is transitory.

Sherrington (1894) long ago observed that when an eye moves in a specific direction, the agonist contracts and the direct antagonist muscle relaxes. When the right eye moves to the left, the right medial rectus muscle contracts and its antagonist the right lateral rectus muscle relaxes. This is Sherrington Law of reciprocal innervation which is both physiologically and clinically important. It explains why squint occurs following paralysis of an extraocular muscle. It has also to be taken care of when surgery on the extraocular muscle is undertaken. Obviously a central innervation causes this kind of version movement.

Hering (1868) vide his "Law of motor correspondence" pointed out that the amount of innervation of the right medial rectus is exactly equal to the amount of innervation of the left lateral rectus and that the inhibitory response to the right lateral rectus is exactly the same as that to the left medial rectus. Herring called these as yoke muscles and the law of reciprocal innervation is known as Herring's law. Thus, the left superior rectus is the yoke muscle of the right inferior oblique and, the right superior rectus is the yoke muscle of the left inferior oblique, the right superior oblique is the yoke muscle of left inferior rectus and similarly the left superior oblique is the yoke muscle to the right inferior rectus muscle.

Primary and Secondary Deviation

If a patient with a paralysed extrinsic ocular muscle is asked to look at a fixation object, he would usually fix the object with the unaffected sound eye and the paralysed eye undergoes deviation. This is the primary deviation. On the other hand, if he is made to fix the object with his paretic eye, the deviation which occurs of the sound unaffected eye is called the secondary deviation (Figs 2.4

and 2.5). If a careful observation is made, it is always found that in a case of recent ocular palsy, the primary deviation of the paralysed eye is less than the secondary deviation of the normal eye. This is because of the fact that when an extrinsic ocular muscle is paralysed, the contralateral synergist overacts. Thus in paralysis of right lateral rectus when right eye fixes an object, the left eye becomes abducted because of overeaction of the left medial rectus. This difference between a primary and secondary deviation tends to disappear in an ocular palsy of long standing.

When considering vertical movements, they are movements of elevation and depression—straight up or straight down. In additions we have elevation in laevoversion that is elevation up and out to the left and elevation up and out to the right (dextroelevation). Similarly depression or downwards movements can be depression of the eye down and out to the left (laevodepression) and depression of the eye down and out to the right (dextrodepression).

In each of these movements, two vertically acting muscles are involved and sometimes it may be difficult to decide which muscle is primarily at fault (or paralysed) specially in long standing cases.

Bielschowsky's head tilting test is of value in differentiating a recent or old paralysis of an oblique from that of a vertical rectus muscle (see Fig. 14.3 in Chapter 14).

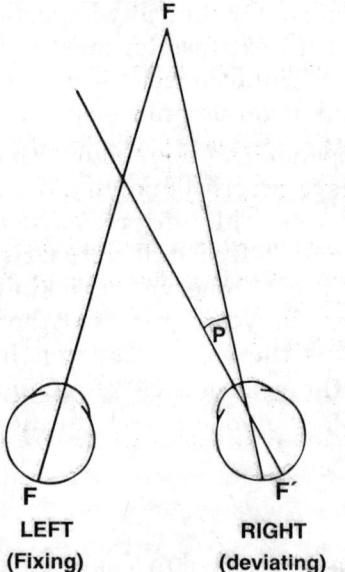

Fig. 2.4: *In noncomitant squint due to recent palsy, P indicates the primary deviation of the affected right eye.*

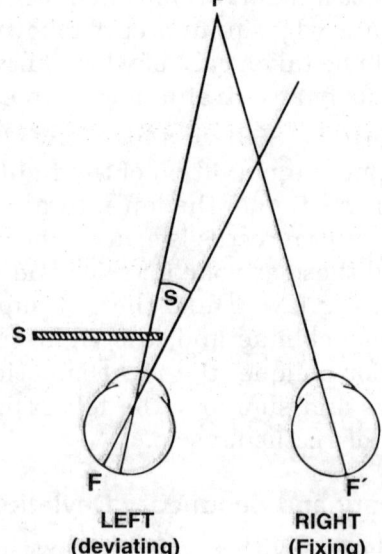

Fig. 2.5: *Indicates the secondary deviation S when the sound nondeviating left eye is occluded by screen* **s***. It would appear that angle P is less than angle S.*

In a case of superior oblique (SO) palsy, the head is tilted to the sound side to compensate the diplopia (in RSO palsy the head is tilted to the left shoulder). If the head is forcibly tilted to the right side (same side as the palsy) as in this case, the eye is intorted by the superior rectus, and the affected right eye moves sharply upwards and the diplopia increases; whereas if on forceful tilting to the paralysed side, the affected right eye does not move or rather moves downwards, it is the superior rectus at fault. However, it must be kept in mind that owing to the development of sequale and of concomitance, this test is not always reliable in the case of a congenital ocular palsy, specially in an adult.

Vergence

The two movements of vergence are convergence and divergence. Convergence occurs when an object approaches the eye and divergence occurs when an object recedes. These movements align the eye in a way which ensures and maintains binocular fixation and binocular vision. In heterophoria (or latent squint) compensatory vergence impulses adjust the tonus of the extraocular muscles to ensure proper relative positioning of the eye. This is necessary for fusion otherwise diplopia may be complained of instead of single binocular vision.

These vergence movements are examples of psychoptical reflexes and the stimulus eliciting the reflex is disparate retinal imagery. Convergence, however, can also be elicited voluntarily.

The nature of divergence and its very existence as a separate reflex function has been questioned. But by and large, it is now accepted as a separate reflex responsible for the eyes to diverge their axes beyond parallelism in distant fixation and presence of divergence excess in clinical practice as divergence excess type of divergent strabismus.

When a retinal image that falls on corresponding retinal elements is shifted so as to fall on disparate retinal elements as is the case with an approaching or receding object or when prisms are placed before the eye, the eyes move to correct their relative position and again bring the images on corresponding retinal areas. This avoids diplopia caused by disparate retinal imagery and ensures bifoveal fixation. However, to produce fusional movements, the disparity must exceed the size of the Panum's area (from Noorden, V.: *Binocular Vision and Ocular Motility,* 4th edn).

In normal individuals, the amplitude of convergence varies from individual to individual depending to a large extent on the state of the individual's neuromuscular apparatus as also whether the individual is being examined when rested or tired or under the influence of a toxic agent.

The amount of convergence and divergence provides information about the patient's ability to cope with a deviation and is also helpful in establishing the type of deviation.

The measurement is in prism-dioptre using a prism (see chapter 4). The patient is comfortably seated and asked to fixate an object. A rotatory or hand-held prism is placed in front of one eye to produce fusional movement. The strength of the prism is increased slowly and stepwise. The patient is asked to report as soon as the fixation object appears double. The required amount of prism strength is gradually reduced and the point at which the fixation object appears again as one single is noted. It is recovery point.

In between is the blur point, that is the point when the fixation object starts becoming blurred as we are increasing the prism strength. This measures the limit within which accommodation can clear the image of the fixation point in spite of increased convergence. And the amount of fusional convergence which is exercised between the blur point and break point represents the absolute convergence.

An examination in the following order serves best to measure both the amount of convergence and divergence. Start with increasing amount of prism base out (this measures convergence). Vergence measurement when measured with a major amblyoscope correspond to those obtained with a rotary prism. Another prism base-in is used to know the limit of divergence exercisable. Then we place the prism base upto to know the downward vergence amount and finally placing the prism base down measures the upward vergence.

Convergence and divergence should always be tested both in distance and near fixation. In patients who complain of difficulties in close work (specially when suspecting a convergence insufficiency) a comparison of the convergence/divergence in distance and near fixation clinches the diagnostic issue.

But what are the normal limits of these vergence movements is rather difficult to quantify. Convergence normally is larger than divergence and vertical vergences are smaller than these. Thus, one set of figures for distance-fixation in an adult is as follows.

Convergence as 20° in each eye divergence as 2° in each eye and sursumvergence and deosunvergence as 3° to 4°.

These measurements for near fixation are greater than the ones mentioned for distance fixation. It should be noted that the amplitude of the vergence varies considerably from one person to another even when function of the binocular system is normal, and more so when the size (linear and vertical) of the fixation objects used for measuring these is variable. They are smallest when fixating light is seen in a completely dark room.

REFERENCES

1. Boeder, P.: An analysis of the general type of Ocular rotations. *Arch Ophthalmol.* 57: 2001, 1957.
2. Boeder, P.: Cooperative actions of extraocular muscle. *Br. J. Ophthalmol.* 46: 397, 1962.
3. Breinin, G. M.: The nature of vergence revealed by electromyography. *Arch. Ophthalmol.* 54: 107, 1955.

4. Breinin, G. M.: The structure and function of the extraocular muscle: An appraisal of duality concept. The Gifford Memorial Lecture. *Am. J. Ophthalmol.* 72, 1. 1971.
5. Duke-Elder, S.: *Textbook of Ophthalmology*, Vol. 1. St. Louis, The C. V. Mosby Co., 1932. reprinted 1946, p. 599.
6. Hyde, J. E.: Some characteristic of voluntary ocular movements in the horizontal plane. *Am. J. Ophthalmol.* 48: 85, 1959.
7. Jampel, R.S.: The fundamental principle of the action of the oblique muscle. *Am. J. Ophthalmol.* 69: 623, 1970.
8. Lancaster, W. B.: Terminology in ocular motility and allied subjects. *Am. J. Ophthalmol.* 26: 122, 1943.
9. Lyle, T.K. and Wybar, K.C.: Lyle and Jackson's *Practical Orthoptics in the Treatment of Squint (and other anomalies of binocular vision),* 5th edn. London, H.K. Lewis, 1970, p. 487.
10. Noorden G.K. Von: *Binocular Vision and Ocular Motility*, 4th edn. St. Louis, The C. V. Mosby Co., 1990.
11. Robinson, D. A.: The mechanism of human saccadic eye movements. *J. Physiol.* (Lond), 174: 245, 1964.
12. Robinson, D. A.: The mechanism of human smooth pursuit movements. *J. Physiology*, 180: 569, 1965.
13. Scobee, R.G. and Green, E. L.: A center for ocular divergence, does it exist? *Am. J. Ophthalmol.* 20: 422, 1946.
14. Westheimer, G. and Mitchell, A. M.: Eye movement responses to convergence stimuli. *Am. Ophthalmol.* 55: 848, 1958.

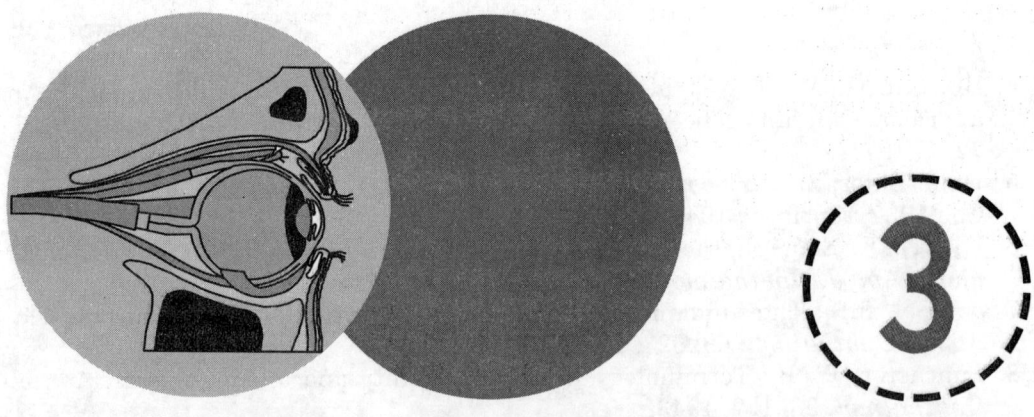

Binocular Single Vision

Binocular single vision (BSV) results from the coordinated use of the two eyes to produce a single mental impression. The images which arise in each of the two eyes separately are appreciated as a single impression in the visual cortex. This cortical integration of similar images on the two retina into a unified perception is binocular single vision (Fig. 3.1).

This faculty of BSV while being an inborn characteristic is potentiated gradually in the first few years of life much the same way as the gradual development of the coordinated use of the arms and legs.

The factors in the successful development and sustenance of BSV are multifactorial—sensory, motor and central. Any obstacle in one or more of these factors (mechanism) could lead to perverse development which in turn would result in ocular deviation or strabismus.

Binocular single vision is a perceptual process of considerable complexity. It has two distinct stages, the presentation of two suitable uniocular sensation contemproneously and the elaboration of these into a unitary perception.

The presence of two uniocular sensations or images on the two retinas (one in each eye) necessitates the following.

1. Overlapping of the visual field of the two eyes so that the same object can be seen by each eye.
2. That corresponding retinocerebral elements are able to function in association with each other, and

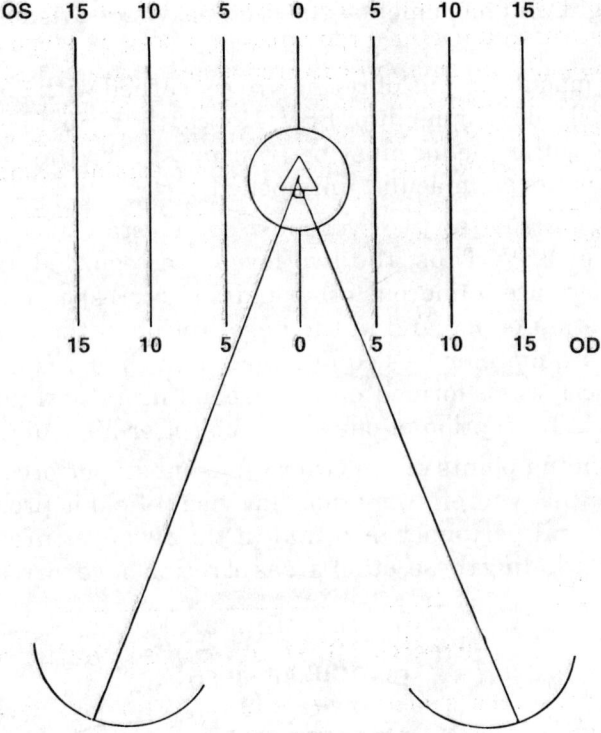

Fig. 3.1: *Single binocular vision; fusion of images from object points.*

3. That the extraocular muscles are able to adjust the visual axis so that corresponding retinocerebral elements are placed in a position to deal with the two images.

The anatomical structures concerned on the sensory side of visual perception or visual impulse are the retinal receptors, the visual pathway up the optic nerve, optic chiasma, optic-tract and optic radiations onto the visual cortex.

Each of these anatomical structures must be healthy so that the visual impulse originating from various retinal receptors (rods and cones) can be easily transmitted to the specified areas of visual cortex for its perception, analysis and coordination with other visual impulses.

Retinal Receptors, their Distribution and Corresponding Retinal Points

Rods and cones are the retinal receptors. Their functional abilities are different. Cones are densely packed in foveal and parafoveal areas to the exclusion of rods and give rise to visual appreciation of form and color—the ingredients of photopic vision (day vision). The rest of the retina has a large number of rods in addition to a small number of cones. They are concerned with the visual appreciation of light and movement—the scotopic vision (vision at night and in dark).

The foveal and macular areas of retina are concerned with good visual acuity which is essential for development of BSV. Hence, they must be fully developed and healthy. The ocular media must be transparent for the visual impulse to pass to these areas (fovea, macula) unimpeded.

The retinal receptors of the two eyes must be in a state of correspondence for the development of BSV. Thus, the two fovea are regarded as corresponding retinal points. There are numerous other pairs of corresponding retinal points in the temporal retina of one and in the nasal retina of the other eye and *vice versa*. And these are more or less equidistant from their respective fovea. The images of the object when formed on corresponding retinal points of the two eyes lead to cortical perception of one single object or binocular single vision.

These corresponding points of the two retinas must, perforce be restricted to the parts of the retina wherein the binocular visual field is projected (Fig. 3.2). The extreme temporal periphery of retina in the two eyes are concerned with uniocular vision. Excluding these, other areas of retina have corresponding retinal

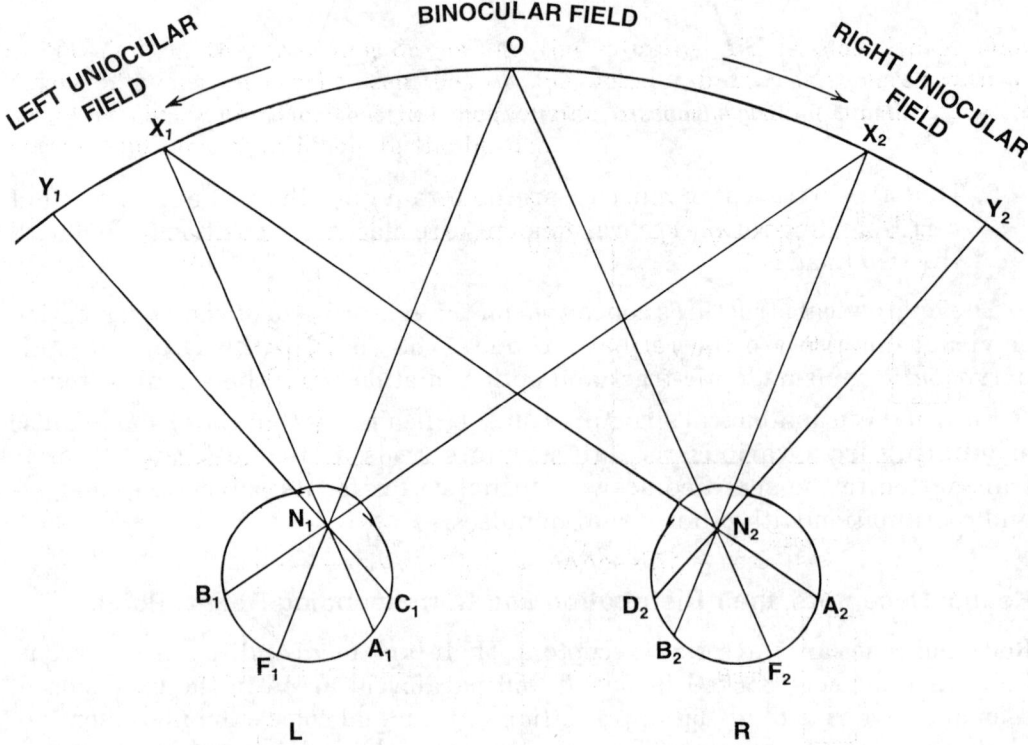

Fig. 3.2: *Visual field—binocular and uniocular field from extreme peripheral parts of retina.*

points and take part in binocular single vision. Any two points which are at equal distance in the same direction from the apparently horizontal and apparently vertical corresponding lines are a pair of corresponding retinal points, viz. the nasal retina of one eye being referred to the temporal retina of the other.

The receptor cells in any small area of one retina correspond to the receptor cells within an equivalent small area in the retina of the other eye. These areas of corresponding retinal points are termed Panum's circle. Each retina contains many such areas and the locus of all object points in space, the images of which fall on these corresponding retinal areas is called the 'horopter', which represents an imaginary surface passing through the points of intersection of the two visual axes.

HOROPTER

In general the horizontal horopter forms a variable line, its form depending on the distance of the point of fixation from the eye (Fig. 3.3 A). Thus, at a distance of nearly two metres it forms (theoretically) a straight line passing through the fixation-points. When the fixation-point is nearer than 2 metres, the locus has its concavity directed to the face. And beyond two metres it forms a convex curve to the face (Fig. 3.3 B).

Panum's Area of Single Binocular Vision

The Danish physiologist Panum first reported that there exists an area around the horopter, stimulation of retinal elements inside which transmits the

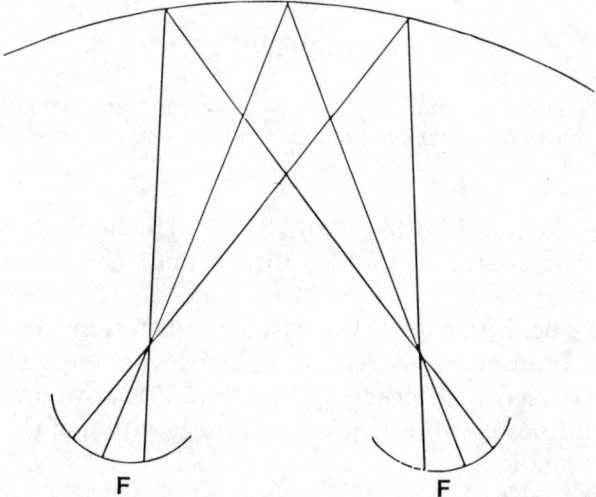

F   F

Fig. 3.3 A: *Horopter. A horopter is an infinitely thin plane drawn through all object points that project on corresponding retinal points.*

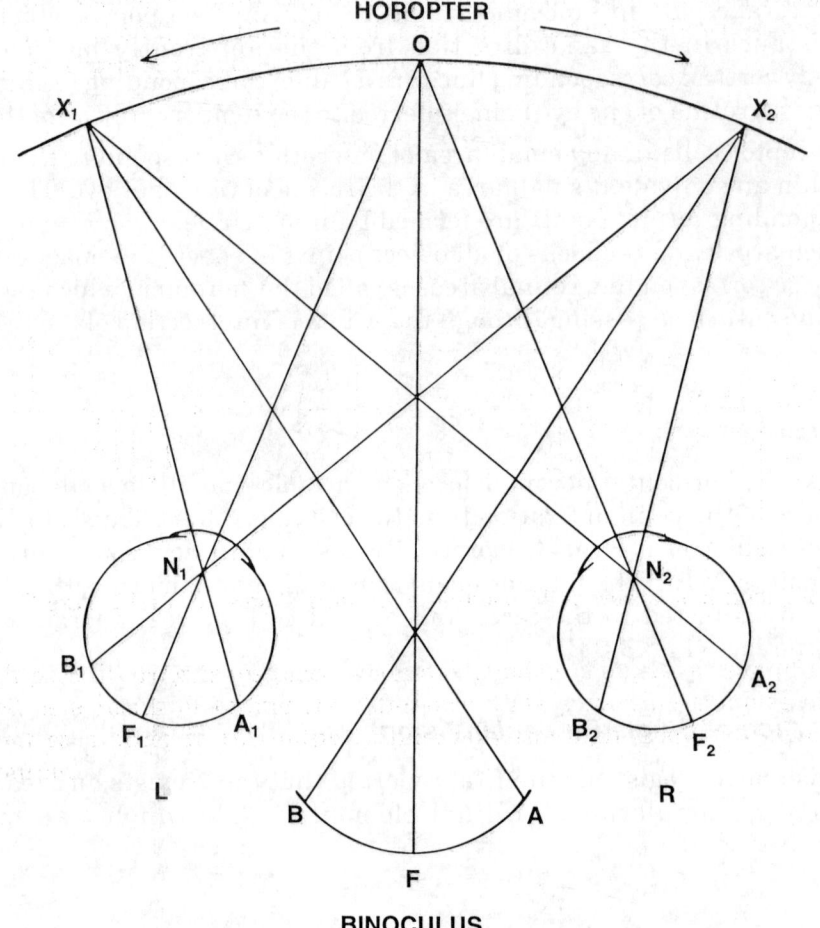

Fig. 3.3 B: *Horopter showing 'binoculus'. Any point on horopter stimulates corresponding retinal points. These corresponding retinal points are represented on binoculus.*

impression of single vision (Figs 3.4 A and 3.4 B). The horizontal extent of these areas is small at the centre (6 to 10 minutes near the fovea) and increases towards the periphery (around 30 to 44 minutes at 12° from the fovea). The vertical extent has been variously assessed by different observers. Volkman (1859) thought the Panum's area is elliptical with the long axis horizontal and which could be increased with practice. Ogle[6] (1950) showed that the length of the axis varies in different subjects and with the position of the retina at which measurements are made.

Whether this Panum's area is in physical space outside the eye or in the retina? This question needs a clear understanding. To quote Von Noorden[9] from his book *Binocular Vision and Ocular Motility*, this area represents the subjective

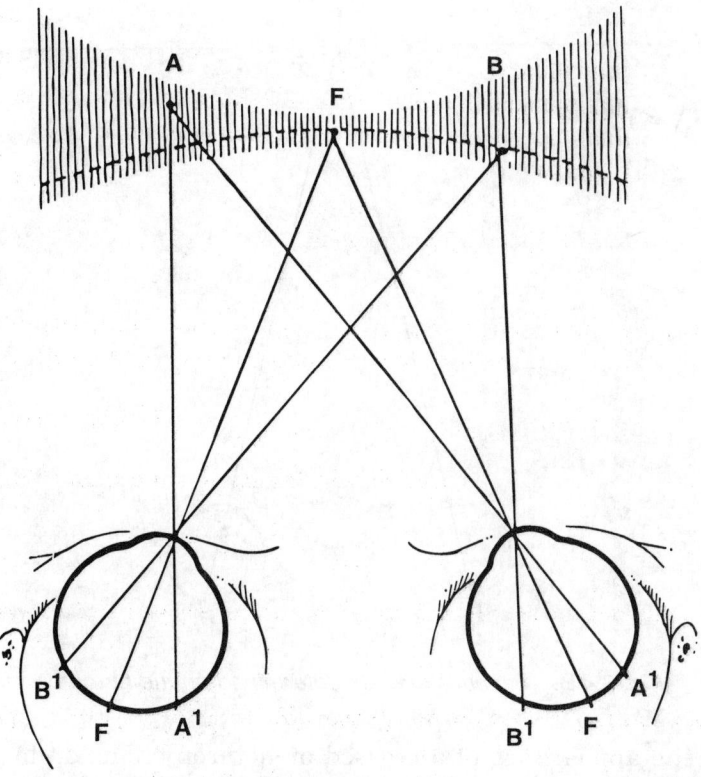

Fig. 3.4 A: *Horopter and Panum's fusional area. Point A is off the horopter but within Panum's area (lined area). It is seen singly but recognised as being further from the observer than points F and B because it is imaged on slightly disparate retinal areas. (This is depth perception on the basis of binocular vision and is called stereopsis.)*

response to a specific stimulus situation eliciting single visual impression. The areas in physical space (location of object points and their images on the retina) simply define operationally the regions within which binocular single vision may be obtained with stimulation of disparate retinal areas.

Simultaneous stimulation of horizontally disparate retinal elements (provided the fused image or the stimulated retinal elements lie within the Panum's area) results in a single visual impression along with depth perception, or *stereoscopic vision* (which is an important ingredient of BSV). On the other hand, vertical displacement produces no stereoscopic effect.

An object which does not lie on the horopter forms images on non-corresponding retinal points and if the attention is drawn, the object appears double. This has been termed physiological diplopia. An object nearer the eye than the fixation object forms images on non corresponding retinal areas and

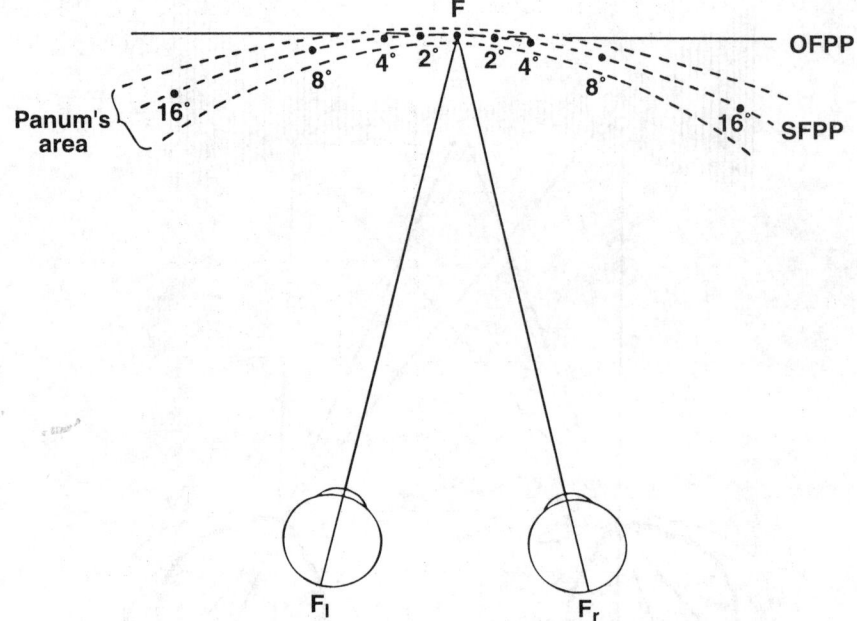

Fig. 3.4 B: *Panum's area as determined on the horopter.*

gives rise to the appearance of a crossed or heteronymous diplopia (Fig. 3.5), whereas when the same object is placed at a distance greater than the fixation object, it produces or gives rise to the appearance of a homonymous or uncrossed diplopia (Fig. 3.6). This physiological diplopia, crossed or uncrossed, seldom obtrudes into consciousness because of a process of neglect or suppression in the visual cortex of all objects which do not lie on the horopter.

It has, however, to be understood that this correspondence of retinal points is not an anatomical peculiarity, but a functional attribute. It is not rigidly determined and is capable of alteration. The development of false macula in a squinting eye which establishes physiological association with the true macula of the other eye is an example of this. After the operation to rectify the deviation or squint, the child may continue to use the false macula preferentially and may be annoyed by double images till a new set of corresponding retinal points is established when the normal macula to macula coordination becomes operative once again.

Suppression

From the moment binocular single vision is established, we learn to disregard the physiological diplopia and unless some abnormal process interferes, we are never aware of it. In acute lateral rectus paralysis of one eye, the affected eye turns in. The patient experiences uncrossed or same sided diplopia (homonymous

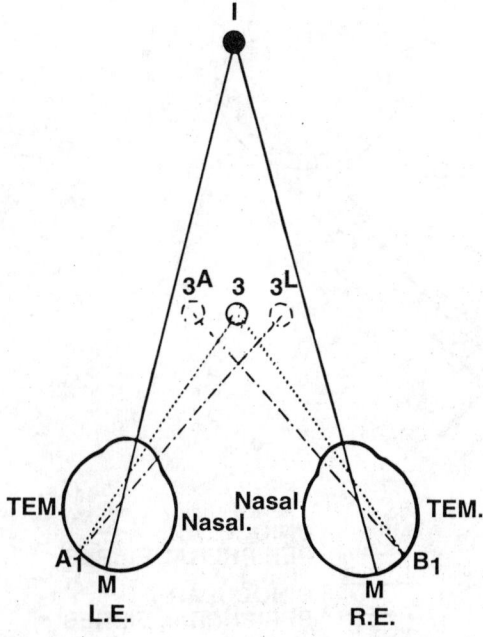

Fig. 3.5: *Diplopia—crossed physiological. Crossed (heteronymous) diplopia of the object P, closer than the fixation point F.*

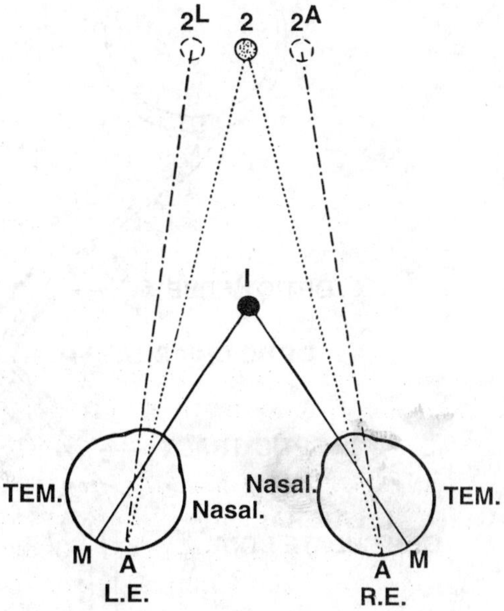

Fig. 3.6: *Diplopia—uncrossed physiological. Uncrossed (homonymous) diplopia of the object P, more distant than the fixation point F, imaged in nasal disparity.*

diplopia). On the other hand, with medial rectus palsy he experiences a crossed diplopia. This is a normal response of the sensory system in course of time. However, by the process of suppression, the unwanted image may be or is ignored by the brain and the diplopia is gone.

Visual impulses or images from the two retinas travel up the corresponding optic nerve. The development of binocular single vision (BSV) is dependent on a hemidecussation of the afferent optic fibres at the chiasma. This enables nerve fibres from corresponding retinal areas of the two eyes to become associated with one another ultimately in the visual cortex (occipital areas of the brain) as shown in Fig. 3.7.

From the functional point of view, each retina may be divided into two halves, the temporal and nasal by a vertical line passing through the centre of fovea. Fibres from the temporal half of the retina including the temporal half of the fovea pass through the optic chiasma without any decussation so that they enter the ipsilateral optic tract. On the other hand, all retinal fibres from the nasal half of the retina including nasal half of the fovea decussate in the chiasma and pass to the contralateral optic tract. Thus, fibres from the temporal retina of one eye (RE) and nasal retina of the other eye (LE) travel in the right optic tract and same sided lateral geniculate body.

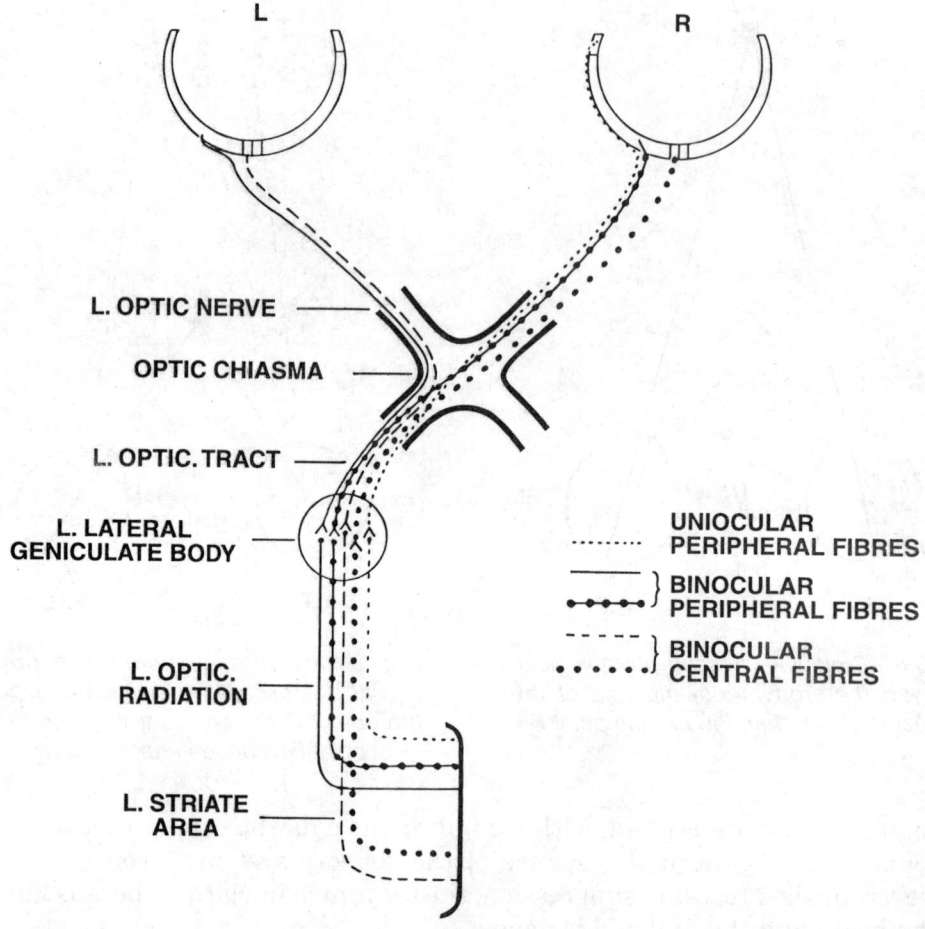

Fig. 3.7: *Afferent visual pathway (from Wolf's Anatomy of Eye).*

Thereafter, they are relayed to the optic radiation and on to the striate-calcarine visual area of the occipital cortex. A few fibres in the afferent visual pathway which are of a non-corresponding nature do not influence the perception of binocular single vision to any significant degree because they are concerned only with a small area of the most peripheral visual field of each eye.

Efferent or Motor Mechanism of BSV (Motor-Fusion)

A successful BSV to be attained and sustained, demands a mechanism of extreme exactitude. This is available to ensure that as far as possible, the two eyes move as a unity preserving a mutual relationship to each other in all positions so that the two images of an object fixated fall upon corresponding points of the two retina. These factors are both anatomical and physiological.

Anatomical factors for binocular single vision are the structure of the bony orbits and their contents. This can be seen in some case of oxycephaly where developmental factors lead to divergence of the bony orbits as also causing exophoria (sometimes). Again, an increase of contents in one bony orbit (fat or growth) may cause the visual axis of the two eyes to be thrown out of alignment, which in turns leads to diplopia.

However, it is the physiological factor, which is more concerned with motor fusion or maintenance of the two eyes in a correct positional relationship both at rest and during movements. Such factors are (1) fixation and re-fixation reflexes and (2) kinetic reflexes.

Fixation and Re-fixation Reflexes

The fixation reflex is present at birth and is initiated by afferent visual stimuli. The presence of an adequately functional fovea is necessary for the fixation reflex. But more than that, the fixation reflex is dependent on the possession by each retinal receptor of a visual spatial or space sense which is distinct from its visual acuity value.

Each retinal receptor possesses a 'local-sign', a term which implies that excitation of a receptor is appreciated in the visual cortex not only in terms of vision but also in terms of projection in space.

In the normal eye, the fovea is highly endowed with local sign and its spatial or space sense consists of a straight-ahead type of projection in the line of fixation. The other retinal receptors are projected on either side of the foveal projection. Receptors near the fovea are projected to the more central part of the visual field and receptors away for the fovea are projected to the more peripheral part of the visual field with the fovea as the central point of reference.

Refixation reflex: It follows shortly after the development of fixation reflex and is concerned with the ability of the eyes to retain fixation of a moving object or to change fixation from one object to another object.

Conjugate fixation reflex: This is fixation reflex simultaneously of both the eyes (at the same time) so that they retain fixation during the course of conjugate movements. It becomes well established by the age of 6 months. There is another reflex which allows the eyes to retain fixation during the conduct of a disjunctive movement and develops at the same time as the conjugate fixation reflex. This is known as the disconjunctival fixation reflex.

Corrective fusion reflex: This reflex enables the eyes to function binocularly even under conditions of stress. It is an elaboration of the conjugate and disconjugate fixation reflexes. It is fully established around the age of 5 yrs, though it starts functioning to some extent from the first year of life and hence it can be disturbed or disrupted easily till the age of 5 years.

Kinetic Reflexes Concerned with Accommodation and Convergence

The acts of accommodation and convergence, so vital for seeing objects at various distances from the eye and seeing them clearly without stress and strain, are also reflexly governed. The relationship is not fixed and rigid, but varies within certain limits. Each of the component may be exercised alone to a certain extent. An exercise of accommodation is followed by an appropriate degree of convergence (accommodative convergence) and the exercise of convergence is followed by an appropriate degree of accommodation (convergence induced accommodation).

But as mentioned above, this relationship is variable. Thus, we may accommodate without any change in convergence (relative accommodation). Similarly the amount of convergence which may be altered in the absence of any change in accommodation is termed the relative convergence. Both these faculties have a positive as well a negative component and are exercised in the interest of clear and stress-free binocular single vision.

Postural Reflexes

These reflexes are concerned with maintenance of the two eyes in their correct relative position within the orbits so that the visual axis are aligned correctly to one another in spite of the changes in the movement of the head relative to the body and or of the body relative to space (as in movements of acceleration and deceleration).

They are both static and stato-kinetic in nature.

Static Reflexes

An example to quote of this reflex is the passive turning of the head to the right followed by a conjugate movement of the eyes to the left.

Stato-Kinetic Reflexes

The conjugate deviation of the eyes which occurs when there is a sudden movement of the body as in acceleration and deceleration although the position of the head is fixed to the space.

The static reflexes are controlled by the labyrinths (the utricle and saccule), whereas the stato-kinetic reflexes are mediated by the semicircular canals.

The Central Mechanism

A composite picture of any object seen and visualised is built up by the activity of the striate areas of both sides of the brain and the final analysis is implemented by the higher visual centres in the adjacent parastriate and peristriate areas (which serve visuopsychic function) so that a relatively crude visual image of the striate areas is given meaning and is integrated with other sensory modalities and with the reaction of past experience. It is not yet fully understood whether this act has any inborn characteristic or whether it is a purely acquired ability dependent for its development on the facilitation and elaboration of the conditioned binocular reflexes. It is established gradually during the early years of life and is dependent for its continuance on a constant reinforcement of the binocular reflexes

On the Efferent Side

We have centres within the cerebrum, one in each frontal area and one in each cerebral cortex. They are responsible for the highest form of control of ocular movement. And a failure in function of one of these cortical centres results in a defect of a particular type of conjugate or disconjugate movement without necessarily affecting isolated movement. These isolated movements are initiated by lower centre (intermediate centres). They (intermediary centres) are possibly four on each side of the brain stem. There are centres for conjugate lateral movement, centre for conjugate vertical movement, a centre for convergence and a centre for divergence.

Besides, there are three nuclei on each side of the brainstem which are concerned with the direct control of the extrinsic ocular muscles of each eye, viz. a principal lateral nucleus, a central or median nucleus, and an accessory nucleus of Edinger-Westphal.

A Normal Binocular Vision

It is a state wherein the eyes are in a state of perfect ocular muscle balance in the straight ahead primary position and in all positions of binocular gaze involving version or vergence type of movements.

Space Perception

Images on disparate points of two retinas (the points, however, lying within the Panum's circle) give rise to depth perception. A true stereoscopic effect cannot be obtained if the images fall upon corresponding retinal points. The higher the disparity of the two points, the greater is the sense of depth perception, or stereopsis. An end point is reached when the two presentations are so dissimilar that they cannot be perceptually fused. And once this limit is overstepped, dissociation occurs, diplopia is produced and the perception of depth is lost.

The minimum detectable horizontal disparity of the images is a measure of stereoacuity. 14 seconds of an arc is the minimum stereoacuity (Parks). It is most conveniently assessed by polaroid vectographic technique.

REFERENCES

1. Ambrose, P. and Noorden, G. K. Von: Past pointing in concomitant strabismus. *Arch. Ophthalmol.* 94: 1896, 1976.
2. Asher, H.: Suppression theory of binocular vision. *Br. Jour. Ophthalmol.* 47: 37, 1953.
3. Brock, F. W. and Givner, T.: Fixation anomalies in strabismus. *Arch. Ophthalmol.* 47: 775, 1952.
4. Hansen, A. K.: "After-image transfer test" in anomalous retinal correspondence. *Am. Ophthalmol.* 52: 369, 1954.
5. Jaffe, N. S.: Anomalous projection. *Am. J. Ophthalmol.* 36: 829, 1953.
6. Ogle, K. N., Martens, TG and Dyer, J. A: *Oculomotor Imbalance in Binocular Vision and Fixation-disparity. Philadelphia, Lea & Febiger,* p. 292,1967.
7. Rohatgi, J. N.: Binocular single vision in concomitant alternating strabismus. *Proc. 47th All India Ophthalmol. Conf.,* Madras, 1989.
8. Swan, K. C.: False projection in comitant strabismus. *Arch. Ophthalmol.* 73: 189, 1965.
9. Von Noorden, G. K.: "Binocular vision and ocular motility", in *Theory and Management of Strabismus*, 4th edn, C. V. Mosby Co., Missouri, 1990.

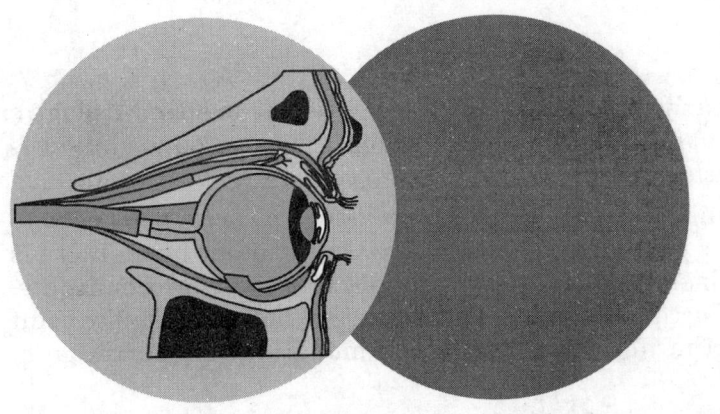
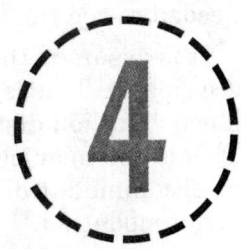

Accommodation–Convergence
State of Convergence and Accommodation

The process whereby the refractive power of the eye is altered to insure a clear retinal image of an object at a particular distance is called *accommodation*. Pari passu there is a change in the inclination of the two visual axes so that the object seen appears as one.

Such a change in the relative position of the two visual axes is called *convergence* when the angle by them (the two visual axes) increases. And is labelled as divergence when this angle decreases. In addition, when seeing at a near distance, the pupil constricts. This triad of accommodation and convergence along with pupillary constriction is the near vision complex. Each of these functions, convergence and divergence, can be dissociated from one another.

ACCOMMODATION

The stimulus to accommodation is a blurred retinal image.

To see an object clearly at a distance of one metre, an emmetrope has to increase the refractive power of the eye by one dioptre. He spends one dioptre of accommodation. Accommodation in dioptre is reciprocal of the distance in metres.

Thus, to see an object clearly at a distance of 50 cm, one has to spend 2 dioptre of accommodation; and at 33.3 cm distance, 3 dioptres of accommodation is needed to see the object clearly.

It is assumed that at infinity an emmetropic eye needs no accommodation to see clearly. This is the far point of accommodation. On the other hand, there is a near fixation distance inside which the eyes cannot effectively accommodate. This is the near point of accommodation. The difference between the far point of accommodation and the near point of (accommodation) is the range of accommodation.

As age advances: Accommodation decreases gradually with the advancing age (Fig. 4.1). This is evident around the age of 40 years when one becomes presbyopic and needs a reading correction. A child of 7 to 8 years of age has an accommodation of 13 to 14 dioptre. It comes down to 3 to 4 dioptre by the age of 40 years and has to be supplemented for reading or seeing at the near distance without any strain.

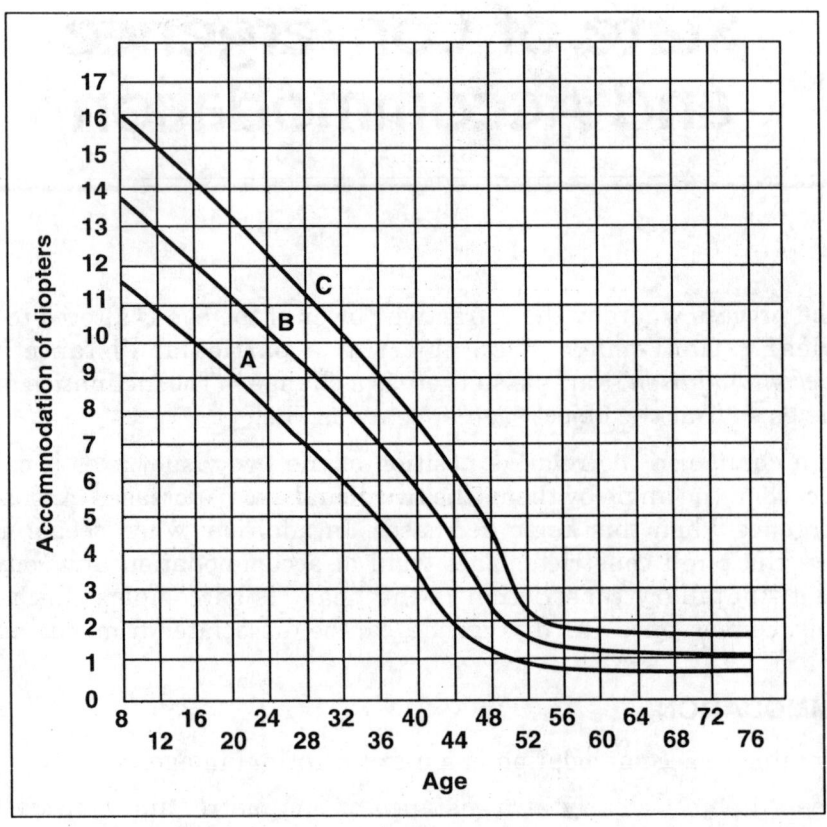

Fig. 4.1: *Age-related standard accommodation Curve in dioptre (from Duane. A., Am J. Ophthal. 5: 865, 1922)*

CONVERGENCE

In order to obtain clear binocular single vision of an object situated at a distance of one metre, not only the eyes have to accommodate but both of these must turn inwards or converge. And the angle through which the two visual axes converge (in the interest of binocular single vision) is called the metre angle (Fig. 4.2).

For objects at one metre distance, convergence of the eyes (the visual axes) required is one metre angle (MA). At a distance of 1/2 metre it is 2 metre angle and at a distance of 1/3 metre it has to be 3 metre angle of convergence (Fig. 4.3).

The metre angle (MA) is a convenient unit since it relates convergence numerically to accommodation. It has to be appreciated, however, that the amount of convergence would be greater, the larger the interocular or interpupillary distance separation. Thus, for an identical metre angle, the amount of needed convergence varies for different individuals.

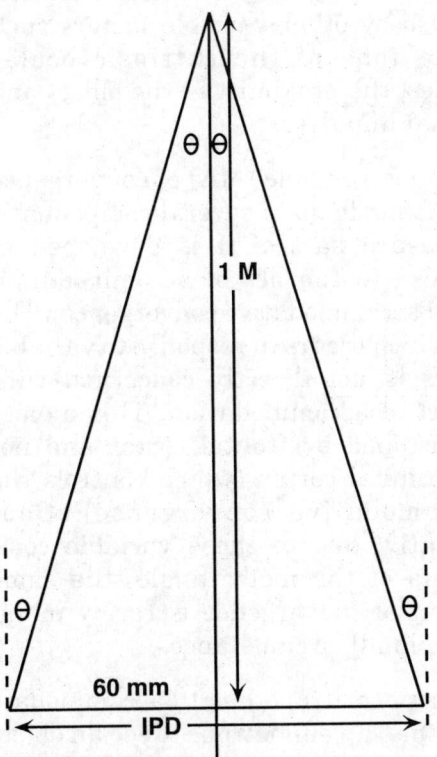

Fig. 4.2: *Metre angle formed by the convergence of the eye to an object situated at one meter distance. IPD = 60 mm.*

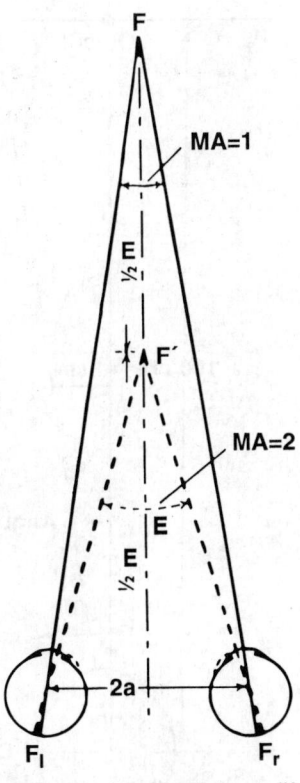

Fig. 4.3: *Metre angle at different distances. 1 MA at one metre distance and 2 MA at ½ metre distance.*

In Clinical Practice

Convergence is measured in prism dioptre (Fig. 4.4). One prism-dioptre displaces the visual axes by 1 cm at a distance of one metre. Thus, if a person converges by 1 cm at one metre distance and has an interocular separation of 6 cm (interpupillary distance), the convergence he must exert is 6.0 prism dioptre. When the same object is fixed at 1/3 metre (33 cm) for the same interocular (interpupillary distance) distance of 6.0 cm the amount of convergence would be 18 prism dioptre or PD.

In clinical practice, the interocular distance—the distance between the centre of rotation of the two eyes—is taken as equivalent to interpupillary distance which is easy to measure. Thus, the amount of convergence is = 1 PD/F where F is the fixation distance in metres.

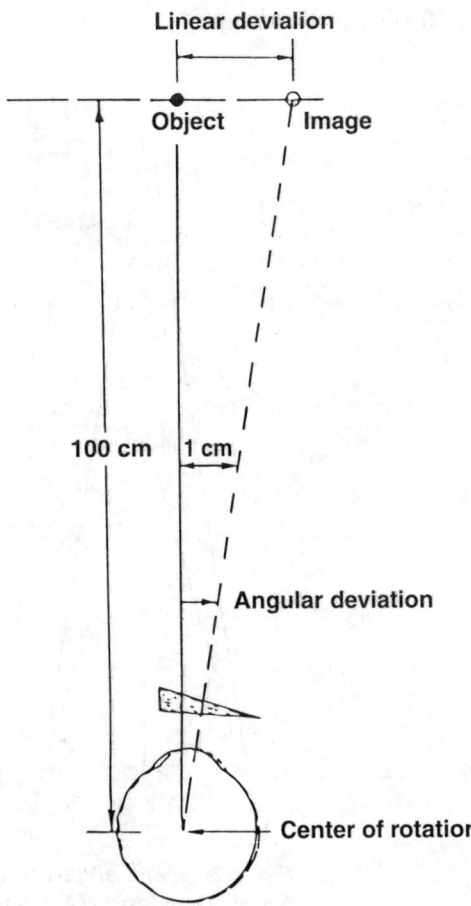

Linear devialion

Object   **Image**

100 cm   **1 cm**

Angular deviation

Center of rotation

Fig. 4.4: *Prism-dioptre definition.*

Every effort of accommodation calls for a convergence response. Under normal conditions of seeing convergence is influenced not only by accommodation but also by other variable factors such as the tone of the extrinsic ocular muscles, the proximity of the object and fusional impulses.

The metre angle (MA) of convergence thus, is made up of several components. A measure part of it is developed in response to the act of accommodation (called accommodative convergence). The part which occurs in response to variable factors is not directly concerned with the act of accommodation. This moiety is controlled by frontal cortex and not the occipital cortex (which controls the accommodative convergence). Consequently, due to these variable components of the metre angle, the same amount of convergence is rarely maintained in all circumstances.

A hypermetrope has to accommodate more than an emmetrope to see an object clearly at one metre and yet the visual axes must not converge more than one metre angle (MA) to maintain clear binocular single vision.

Existence of a central mechanism for convergence and possibly of a divergence is thus called forth. This arises in frontal cortex.

Involuntary convergence is a psychooptical reflex based upon fixation and refixation reflexes. Even though it occurs reflexly without volition, it is dependent upon the perceptual appreciation of fixation and requires the active intervention of attention. It is a fusion movement that is constantly being employed.

Reflex Convergence or Involuntary Convergence

This can be of the following types:

1. Accommodative convergence,
2. Proximal convergence,
3. Tonic convergence, and
4. Fusional convergence.

According to some authors, there is also a voluntary component of convergence in which no external stimulus is needed to exercise convergence. A child can converge his eyes seemingly at will without exercising any accommodation (a voluntary squint in a child). This, however, is not acceptable to Jampolsky and others.

The usual position of rest for the eyes is one of slight divergence and hence, a moiety of convergence is required constantly to maintain parallelism of the eyes in the primary position (tonic convergence).

The total excursion from the position of rest has three components of convergence—tonic, accommodative and fusional. Proximal convergence is induced by the awareness of nearness of an object. This may be either an object at near vision distance or one though situated at near vision distance has been optically placed at infinity such as what happens in a major amblyoscope.

Tonic convergence is mediated by the tone of the ciliary muscle and is of a static nature. As the fixation object comes closer to the near point, convergence is increasingly employed synergically with accommodation, the stimulus for fusion adding considerably to it total amplitude. The extent of this reflex moiety is seen when fusion is suddenly abolished at the near point by occluding one eye, whereupon the covered eye deviates outwards.

Although for analytical reason, both physiological and clinical, it is necessary to separate the various components of a convergence movement, but convergence is a unitary process. The central nervous system arrangements are probably located in the midbrain and have numerous connections with various cortical, subcortical and peripheral retinal areas. And thus, changes in convergence position can be elicited in many different ways.

The main symptom of convergence insufficiency is eyestrain, specially when reading, writing or doing any close work. This is because of blurring and sometimes diplopia. To continue (doing) the near-work results in headache and the work may be given up as happens to students at the time of examination when the continuous study for hours together tires the extraocular muscles as also the ciliary muscles (which are constantly at work to provide accommodation).

If a psychogenic factor is superadded, as happens on these occasions, symptoms of eyestrain are aggravated. The symptoms are varied in their incidence. However, many cases suffer no discomfort.

Diagnosis of convergence insufficiency is usually easy. The ocular movements are full and normal. The eyes fail to converge fully on looking at a near object when one eye only appears to take up fixation.

In these cases of convergence insufficiency muscle-balance testing reveals the following.

1. Maddox-Rod reading at the distance of 6 metres as normal or orthophoric.
2. Whereas with Maddox wing examination at 33 cm there is exophoria of 6 Δ or more, and
3. The near point of convergence is more than 9.5 cm.

Convergence insufficiency has to be distinguished from exophoria. In exophoria of the basic type, the Maddox rod and Maddox wing readings are more or less equal. In divergence excess type of exophoria on the other hand, the divergence is greater for distance (Maddox rod) and the near point of convergence is normal. The prism-convergence is normal and prisms divergence is abnormal. With these clinical findings one can differentiate between a convergence insufficiency and exophoria.

Relative insufficiency of convergence may result from

1. Anatomical conditions such as a wide interpupillary distance which makes convergence difficult.
2. Delayed development.
3. When the accommodative part of accommodation convergence reflex is not employed as may happen in uncorrected myopia, high hypermetropia and astigmatism (when accommodation is not used rather given up for it fails to make near objects appear clear).
4. General disease or disability as after prolonged illness, and toxic condition, etc.

Treatment

Treatment of convergence insufficiency is satisfactory. The nervous element has to be taken care of. Any physical illness causing general body weakness has to be treated. Refractive error, if any, has to be adequately corrected. Hypermetropes should be given an undercorrection and myopes should be fully corrected.

The role of orthoptic exercises to increase convergence and relax divergence comes thereafter; and finally when that also fails, relieving prism base-in should and could be prescribed in spectacles for near work.

Convergence Excess

1. Associated with an increase in accommodation an increase of convergence is but natural for these two physiological actions are habitually synergic. Thus, in all uncorrected hypermetropic children an excessive accommodation may initiate excess of convergence causing symptom. In poor illumination, after debilitating illness and corneal leucoma, etc., the desire for clear vision leads to accentuated accommodation and this in turn causes convergence excess.
2. A hysterical convergence spasm with miosis and accommodative spasm is not very unusual.

Symptoms of convergence excess: These are annoying. The letters in the book become blurred. Fatigue and headache easily follow continued concentration on near work/reading. This is clearly seen in young adults recovering from a long illness when they quickly give up close work because of undue fatigue and headache resulting from convergence excess.

Treatment The etiological or causative factors should be removed. Refractive error has to be adequately corrected. The amount of near work may have to be reduced till symptoms persist. General health has to be taken care. And finally orthoptic exercise inducing voluntary relaxation is of help.

Fusional Convergence

The eyes are directed to the object of attention and interest and maintained in positions relative to each other so that the images of the object (of fixation) fall on the fovea of each eye simultaneously. This is brought about by fusional convergence reflex.

Any error of ocular alignment caused by the refractive error of the two eyes or by excessive tonic or proximal convergence has to be corrected. And herein, comes the fusional convergence reflex.

Any excess of convergence for ocular alignment is adjusted by inhibition of convergence. So long this excess of convergence falls within the limits of the individual's fusional convergence (till then), the deviation remains latent and clear, and comfortable binocular single vision is maintained.

Accommodational Convergence

Most of the troubles that arise from anomalies in and of convergence occur during near work. Relative convergence is the amount that can be exerted or relaxed while the accommodation is kept constant. This relationship is very elastic.

This relative convergence can be divided into three parts—a positive portion, the middle-third and a negative portion. The positive portion has to be larger than the negative so that there is ample converging power in reserve. It is measured by the strongest adducting prism (prism base-out) which can be tolerated without provoking diplopia (while fixing an object at a particular distance). On the other hand, the strongest prism base-in that can be tolerated without causing diplopia is the negative portion, that is the amount by which convergence can be relaxed.

The middle-third of convergence is the amount which is used for any particular distance of work along with the fixed amount of accommodation for that distance. At the same time a large positive and negative relative accommodation is necessary for comfortable work without causing strain or fatigue of convergence. And in clinical practice a condition of relative insufficiency for the particular working distance employed is more important.

A condition of absolute insufficiency may be said to exist when the near point, in the absence of presbyopia, is greater than 11 cm from the interocular base line (9.5 cm from the apex of the cornea) or when there is difficulty in attaining 30^0 of convergence.

Accommodative Convergence/Accommodation (AC/A) Ratio

When a person exerts a certain amount of accommodation, a determined amount of convergence is brought into play. This is the accommodative-convergence. A normal emmetropic person would be expected to exert 1 MA of convergence for each dioptre of accommodation (or its equivalent in prism dioptre) but this may not always be the case. The response to a unit stimulus of accommodation with a specific amount of convergence may be greater or smaller convergence than is called for by the convergence requirement.

The Ac/A ratio: Fry[5] expresses the ratio of the amount of accommodative-convergence measured (in prism dioptres) to the number of dioptres of accommodation which causes the convergence, other factors causing convergence remaining constant. The average numerical value of this ratio is said to be 3:1 to 5:1 (convergence measurement is related to 1 dioptre of accommodation).

Determination of Ac/A Ratio

A simple comparison of the deviation in distance and near fixation is commonly used in clinical practice to estimate the Ac/A ratio. If the two measurements are equal, the Ac/A ratio is said to be normal. If the near measurement in a esotropic case is greater by 10 Δ or more, the Ac/A ratio is said to be high.

Measurement of Ac/A Ratio by Heterophoria Method

Use is made of the prism and alternate cover method along with the use of a target like Snellen's test type letter (to ensure a steady accommodation both at distance and near) or a Maddox tangent scale. The deviation of the eye is measured in prism dioptre at a distance of 6 metre (optical infinity where no accommodation is presumed to be exerted) and then the deviation is measured at 33 cm (1/3 metre) using a Maddox wing, the point of near fixation assuming again that the convergence exerted is caused wholly by the accommodation synkinesis. When the measurement for distance and near is equal, the Ac/A ratio is normal; when it is greater for distance then for near, the Ac/A ratio is low; and when it is greater for near than for distance, the Ac/A ratio is high.

To give the Ac/A ratio, a precise value by this method, the interpupillary distance (IPD) is measured in cm. In this way

$$\text{Ac/A ratio} = \text{IPD} + \frac{D_2 - D_1}{F_1}$$

IPD = Interpupillary distance in cm

D_2 = Latent deviation for near (1/3 M)

D_1 = Latent deviation for distance (6 M)

F_1 = Fixation distance at near in dioptre that is the amount of accommodation in dioptre exerted at 1/3 metre by an emmetrope, or

F_2 = Distance of near fixation in metre.

Thus when IPD = 6 cm $D_2 = 10\ \Delta$ exo

$D_1 = 4\ \Delta$ exo

$F_1 = 3\ D$ or $F_2 = 1/3\ M.$

$$\text{Ac/A} = 6 + \frac{-10 - (-4)}{3} = 6 + \frac{(-10 + 4)}{3} = 6 + \frac{(-6)}{3} = 6 - 2 = 4$$

Thus the Ac/A ratio equals 4 Δ of accommodative convergence for each dioptre of accommodation. And this is said to be normal.

2. Gradient Method

In this method, the change in stimulus to accommodation is produced by means of ophthalmic lenses and not by change in viewing distance. The distance is fixed, convex (+) lenses by decreasing the amount of accommodation needed for this given distance decrease the amount of convergence and concave (−) lenses by increasing the amount of accommodation increases the amount of convergence for the same distance both for producing clear binocular single vision.

A Maddox rod is placed in front of one eye and correcting prism (a rotating prism) in front of the other eye. This gives the amount of initial deviation eso or exo. Thereafter a convex or concave lens is placed in front of this eye. This placing of lenses induces a change of accommodation and pari passu a change of convergence which is measured by the correcting prism in front of the other eye. Thus, for a given fixation distance the Ac/A ratio is

$$Ac/A = \frac{\Delta^1 - \Delta^0}{D}$$

Where

Δ^0 is the original deviation (eso of exo),

Δ^1 deviation with the spherical lenses (convexs and concave taken together for the fixed distance) and

D   is the fixation distance is dioptre (the power of the lens).

AC   accommodative convergence in prism dioptre and accommodation is in dioptre =

Example

when $\Delta^0 = 2 \Delta$ eso

$\Delta^1 = 6 \Delta$ Eso, D = 1 Disph (– ve lens)

$$Ac/A = \frac{6 - 2}{1} = 4$$

The value for Ac/A ratio by the gradient method is somewhat lower than that obtained by the heterophoria method because the fixed distance which is adopted throughout in the gradient method does not allow for the influence of the factor of proximal convergence. It is entirely the accommodating convergence or the patients subjective accommodative effort.

This gradient method of determining Ac/A ratio can easily be obtained using a major amblyoscope or synoptophore. It is rather more practical to obtain Ac/A ratio in the manner below (gradient method).

On a major amblyoscope, the subjective angle of the deviation is determined as usual, after setting the instrument to the interpupillary distance, using correcting glass power worn by the patient' and using slides to find out foveal fixation. The subjective angle is recorded on the prism-dioptre scale.

After this a concave lens (– 3.00 Dspl) is placed in the lens holder of the instrument (one in front of each eye). This leads to increased accommodation and pari passu increased accommodative convergence to maintain clear foveal fixation. The subjective angle is then determined on the prismdioptre scale.

Ac/A ratio is calculated as follows:

$$Ac/A = \frac{D_2 - D_1}{D}$$

D_1 = subjective angle with patients own glasses.
D_2 = subjective angle with addition of – 3.00 Dspl. and
D = the strength in dioptre of the concave spherical lens used.
If D_2 = 19 Δ Eso
D_1 = 7 Δ Eso
D = – 03.00 Dspl.

$$Ac/A = \frac{19.00 - (+7)}{3} = \frac{12}{3} = 4$$

Treatment and Ac/A Ratio

A normal Ac/A ratio indicates that the amount of convergence is proportional to the amount of accommodation used to correct an uncorrected hypermetrope. But in some cases, the determining factor is an excessively high response of the convergence mechanism to any accommodative effort. With a normal Ac/A ratio one can expect that with the correction of the refractive error, the ocular deviation is normalised whereas with a high Ac/A ratio, this does not happen.

When treating cases of accommodative esotropia or convergent squint cases with miotics (usually phospholine iodide 0.3% solution) there is change in Ac/A relationship. Less of accommodation is needed to see clearly a near object and hence less accommodative convergence effort is brought into play. This reduces the high Ac/A ratio to normal value. Para sympathomimetic drugs affect the pupil reducing the size. The greater depth of focus of an eye with a narrow pupil would reduce the need to accommodate and hence, reduce the accommodative effort and thus would lead to less effort of convergence and thereby reduce the angle of esodeviation.

It has been suggested that a decrease in the effectiveness of the medial rectus muscle by a recession-operation in accommodative esotropia results in a reduction of the value of an abnormally high Ac/A ratio.

REFERENCES

1. Adler, F. H.: *Physiology of the Eye: Clinical Application*, 4th edn. St. Louis, The C. V. Mosby & Co., 1965.
2. Cohen, M. M. and Alpern, M.: Vergence and accommodation–VI. The influence of ethanol on the Ac/A ratio. *Arch. Ophthalmol*. 81: 518, 1969.
3. Dsuane, A: Studies in monocular and binocular accommodation with their clinical applications. *Am J. Ophthalmol* 5: 805, 1922.

4. Franceschetti, A. T. and Burian H. M.: Gradient accommodative convergence — accommodative ratio in families with and without esotropia. *Am. J. Ophthalmol.* 70: 558, 1970.

5. Fry, G. A.: The effect of age on the Ac/A ratio. *Am. J. Ophthalmol.* 36 : 299, 1959.

6. Jampolsky, A.: Ocular divergence mechanism. *Trans. Am. Ophthalmol. Soc.* 68: 730: 1970.

7. Morgan, M. W., Jr.: Relationship between accommodation and convergence. *Arch. Ophthalmol.* 47: 745, 1952.

8. Noorden, G. K. Von, Morris, J. and Edelman P.: Efficacy of bifocals in the treatment of accommodative esotropia. *Am. J. Ophthalmol.* 85 : 830, 1976.

9. Noorden, G. K. Von and Avilla, C. W.: Non-accommodative excess. *Am. J. Ophthalmol.* 101, 70, 1986.

10. Parks, M. M.: Abnormal accommodative convergence in squint. *Am. J. Ophthalmol.* 59 : 364, 1958.

11. Sears, M. and Guber, D.: The change in the stimulus Ac/A ratio after surgery. *Am. J. Ophthalmol.* 64: 872, 1967.

12. Sloan, L., Scar M. L, and Jablonski, M. D.: Convergence-accommodation relationship. *Am. J. Ophthalmol.* 63 : 283, 1960.

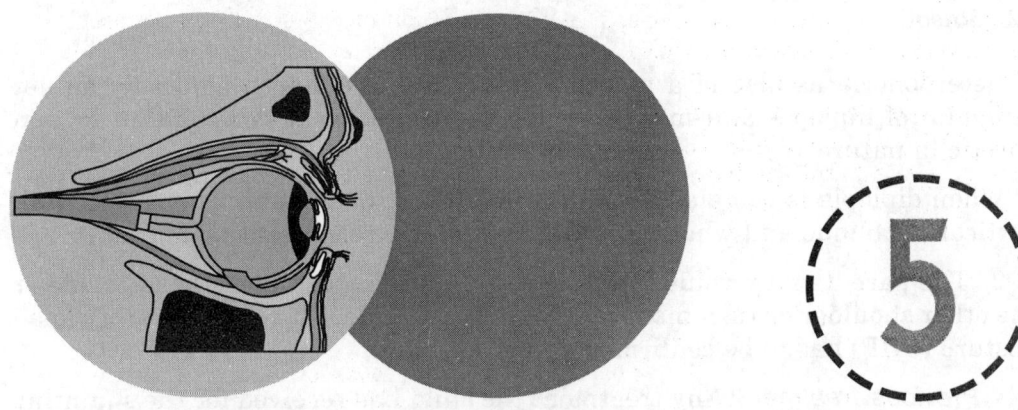

Examination and Investigations

A detailed case history is helpful in diagnosis, prognosis and treatment. In children it has to come from questioning the parents and in adults it has to include information about their work or profession.

- *Case History:* The case history includes the following:

1. The age at which the ocular deviation was first seen or noticed and the age at the time of examination and the start of treatment.

2. Who first noticed the squint: the parents, relations or the family doctor?

3. The nature of the deviation or squint: Does the affected eye turns in, out, up or down or shows a combination of these?

4. Which eye deviates: Right or left, or is it alternating, that is sometimes the left eye turns and sometimes the right eye turns?

5. Was the onset of the deviation sudden, gradual or intermittent?

6. Is the deviation constant or intermittent? If constant, did it start as constant or was it preceded by a period of intermittency?

- *Other Disorders* 1. Any illness at the time of onset of squint? In a number of children deviation of the eye follows illness such as whooping cough, measles and debilitating illness, etc. Parents often lay emphasis on this point saying the eyes were alright before and have started deviating after the febrile illness. 2. Following head injury, some children may develop squint which is generally paretic in nature.

- *Symptomatology* 1. Some patients, specially youngsters, complain of seeing double or diplopia looking straight ahead or on moving the eye. This is a feature of heterophoria as also of a paretic squint. Young children generally do not complain of diplopia and more so when the deviation is concomitant or non paretic in nature.

When diplopia is complained of, one has to ask for its nature — horizontal, vertical or oblique and whether it is constant or intermittent in character.

2. The parents may volunteer that the child likes to tilt his head to one or the other shoulder or turn his face to right or left side. This compensatory head posture (CHP) has to be confirmed on examination.

• *Previous Treatment:* Any treatment the child has received for the squinting eye. This may be glasses for the refractive error or occlusion of the good eye or operation on the deviating eye.

• *Family History:* Any family history of squint in parents or close relations and the nature of treatment undertaken, if any.

Clinical Examination

After a careful case history has been obtained, the ophthalmologist carries out routine clinical examination of the eyes before embarking on special examination and investigations (for the squint).

A look at the patient from top to the toe is necessary. Any facial asymmetry, tilt of the head to one or the other shoulder or turning of the face (compensatory head posture) indicates an associated vertical component in the ocular deviation. Similarly the widening or narrowing of the palpebral aperture gives us some definite information (to be discussed later).

The next is elicitation of ocular movements in all the cardinal directions of conjugate movement-to right (dextroversion) to left (laevoversion) to up and down, up and out to right, down and out to right, up and out to left and down and out to left and finally the eyes looking straight ahead (the primary position).

Any restriction of movement or of deviation in one or more of these cardinal positions would mean that we are dealing with a case of non-comitant squint. In concomitant squint cases, the ocular movements are full and normal in all these directions.

Examination of ocular media and fundus oculi is important in order to eliminate possible ocular causes of defective vision such as corneal-leucoma, lental opacity, other organic diseases of the media, optic atrophy, etc. These may cause a secondary concomitant squint.

The *visual acuity* is carefully recorded (the details of how to do this and more so in young children and infants is described later on).

The next is *refraction*. Refraction has to be assessed under full mydriasis and cycloplegia. For this the time honoured use of atropine sulph eye ointment (1%)

applied twice a day in both the eyes for at least five days. This is essential. To cut the time in number of days the child has to wait, opinion now veers round to using atropine ointment for at least two days and three times a day. Some surgeons prefer to use a mild cycloplegic and mydriatic like cyclopentolate 1% or tropicamide 1% (two to three instillations in 1/2 to one hour). Thereafter, retinoscopy is carried out, full refractive error is assessed and correcting lens prescribed. The correction in a hypermetropic or astigmatic refraction should be full as per the retinoscopic finding. The astigmatic correction has to be prescribed in full whereas, for high hypermetropia it may not be full or total correction if this is going to be uncomfortable to the child.

Some children are not able to relax accommodation (when hypermetropia is corrected for the first time) and complain of blurring of distance vision. To avoid this, it is suggested that parents be advised to get the prescribed glasses immediately within a day or two and insist the child to use the glasses while the effect of atropine ointment (relaxation of accommodation) is still on. This has been found to facilitate acceptance of the correcting glass.

Corrective Lenses Serve Two Useful Purposes

1. They create a sharp retinal image which in young children is essential as a stimulus for the use of the eyes and for fusion, and
2. They assist in producing the proper balance between accommodation and convergence.

Coming Back to Visual Acuity Assessment

1. In infants, if by history and observations one eye is always found to be deviated or when the infant does not like closing the other eye while he has no objection to closing the deviated eye, the assumption of an existing or impending amblyopia in the deviating eye should be made and immediate treatment is called forth.

But to assess the visual acuity in an infant with heterotropia is not an easy task. Three methods available are:

1. Optokinetic nystagmus
2. Preferential looking, and
3. Visual evoked electric potential (EVP) or visual evoked response (VEP).

However, none of these techniques is sufficiently developed for use in routine clinical practice.

In optokinetic nystagmus, a succession of black-and-white strips is passed through the patient's field of vision on a rotating drum. This elicits nystagmus.

The visual angle subtended by the smallest strip width that elicits an eye movement (minimum separable) is a measurement of visual acuity.

Preferential Looking

This technique is based on the fact that an infant's attention is more attracted by patterned stimuli than by a homogenous surface. Hence, if offered the choice between patterned stimuli, say black and white strips, and a homogenous background, an infant will prefer to look at the patterned stimuli as long as the pattern is above the visual acuity threshold. Visual acuity (VA) determined with this method ranges from approximately 6/24 in the newborn to 6/60 at 3 months and 6/6 at 36 months of age.

VEP refers to electrical potentials recorded from the scalp overlying the visual cortex.

A variety of stimuli and recording methods using these cortical potentials have been used to assess visual acuity in infants. Most of these studies suggest that the infant's visual system matures to allow detection of 6/6 targets by the age of one year or possibly earlier.

Visual Acuity (VA) in Pre-School Age Children

The visual acuity in children in the age group of 2 to 3 years can be examined by the following methods.

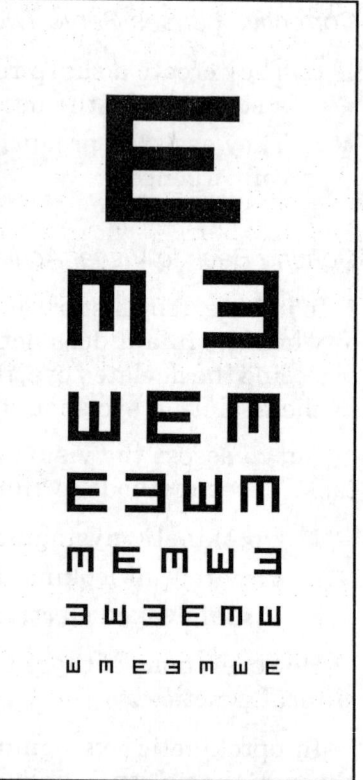

1. *Using an E Test:* It is better to have a rotating E board. The examiner standing at the required distance of 6 metres away from the child holds the board up and rotates the E into various positions while the child with a plastic or wooden E in his hand is instructed to place the E, the same way up, down, sideways as the one to which the examiner is pointing (Figs 5.1 and 5.2). Modifications can be made as desired.

2. *Sheridon-Gardiner test:* It is another useful test for determining the visual acuity in a young child.

3. *Snellen-chart:* This chart with different sizes of the animals (familiar ones) can be shown to a child to assess his VA at distance.

Visual Acuity in School-age Children

To assess the visual acuity in school-going children and in adults, Snellen charts with letters or Landolt ring (broken C) or projection devices

Fig. 5.1: *The E-test for illiterates and young children.*

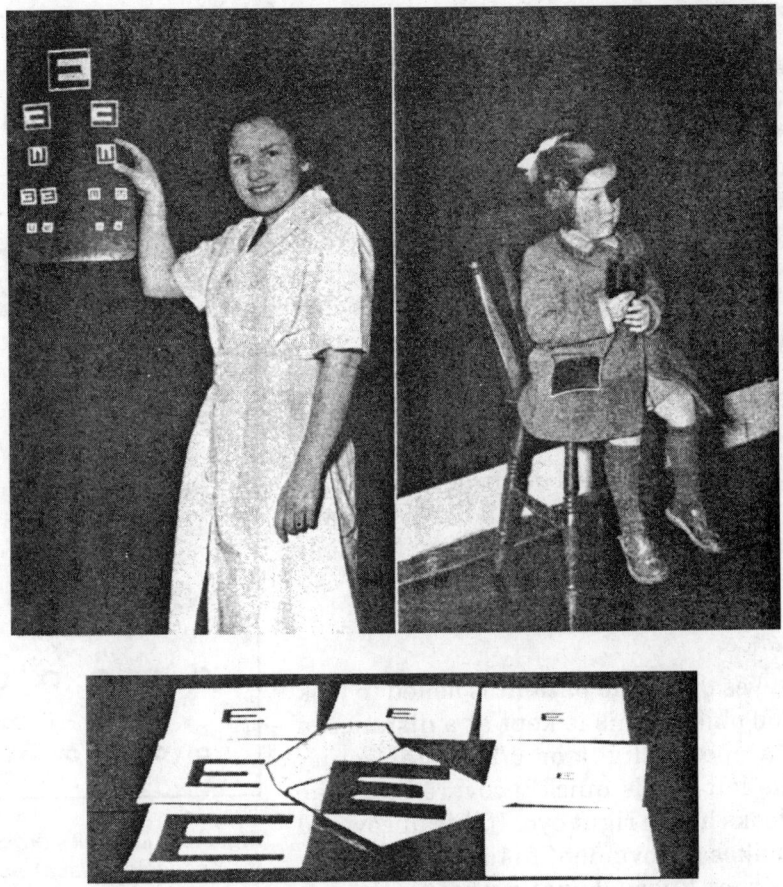

Fig. 5.2: *The examiner placing E (different sizes) in different ways to attract the attention of the child and thereby to have an idea of the visual acuity level.*

can be used to assess the distant visual acuity (Fig. 5.3). Near distance visual acuity can be assessed by graduated reading test types charts.

Observation of the Ocular Posture and Cover Test

It has already been stated that while examining the eyes, attention must be paid to the palperbral aperture and its width. One has to notice whether the width changes when the patient moves the eyes to the right or left as in a retraction syndrome of Duane or when the patient chews as occurs in jaw winking phenomena of Marcus-Gunn.

In infants the epicanthus frequently is more pronounced (a semilunar fold of skin running downward at the site of the nose) and its concavity directed towards the inner canthus. This is a common cause of pseudostrabismus. However, with the growth of nose and face as the age advances, the epicanthic fold recedes.

COVER-TEST

A valuable clinical method of detecting the presence of a manifest or a latent squint is by means of the cover-test[1, 3, 17]. It also tells us the direction of the deviation, the fixation behaviour and (even) whether the visual acuity is significantly reduced in the deviating eye. (This is of great importance in the infant who does not cooperate otherwise). The test can be conducted as follows

The Cover Test to Detect the Presence of a Manifest Strabismus:

Such a test has to be carried out first for distance looking at a spot of light or a small fixation object at a distance of 6 metres and then for near distance (at one-third or half metre).

1. For Distance

With both eyes open, the patient is asked to look on a fixation object. This is kept at a distance of 6 metre—a spot of light or 6/9 visual acuity symbol. His left eye is quickly covered and the examiner looks at the right eye. If this uncovered right eye makes a movement to take up fixation, it indicates that it was deviating before the left eye was covered. A movement outwards of the right eye indicates that it was in a convergent position before and a movement of right eye inwards indicates that it was in divergent position before (Fig. 5.4).

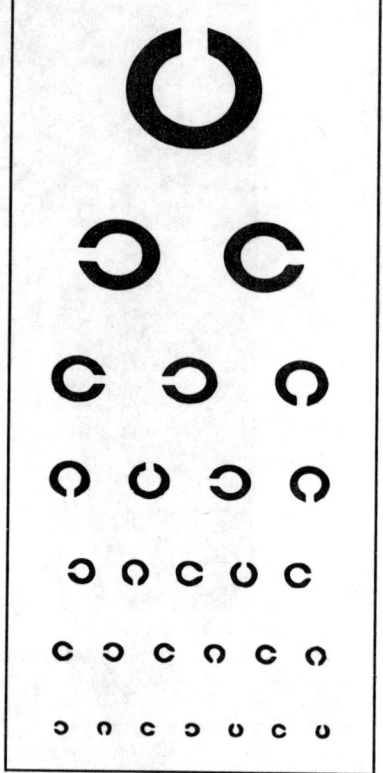

Fig. 5.3: *Landolt's broken ring test for assessing visual acuity in the same way as with E test.*

The cover is then applied to right eye and the left eye is observed for any movement inwards or outwards as above. This procedure should be repeated twice or thrice to ensure a correct observance. No movement in either eye on uncovering and covering indicates no deviation or squint.

2. For Near

The test is carried out in a similar manner using a fixation object held at a distance of one-third or half metre. For young children, a spot light along with a sound producing device is the best to attract attention and fixation.

This Cover-test would then Tell us

 a. A manifest squint for right or left eye or alternating in nature,
 b. The deviation type—convergent, divergent or vertical,

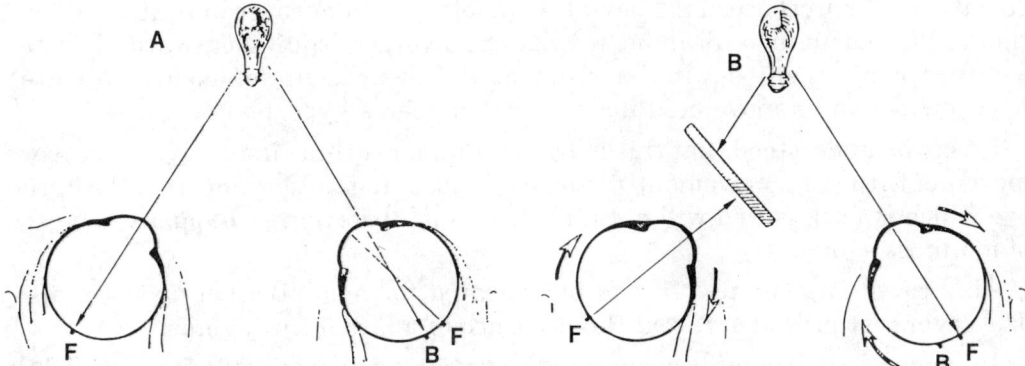

Fig. 5.4: *Cover-test.* **A** *Right eye is turned in (esotropia) and thus while fixing, the image of the light falls on a point B on the nasal side of the right fovea F whereas in the left straight eye it falls on the fovea of the left eye.* **B** *The left eye is covered and the patient is asked to look at the light. Observer notices the right eye moving out to take up fixation so that the image of the light now falls on fovea F of the right eye. This indicates a manifest convergent squint of the right eye.*

    c. Presence of deviation both for distance and near or only for distance or for near, and

    d. The amount of deviation with or without the glasses being used.

However, when the visual acuity is very low the deviating eye does not fix readily or fixes eccentrically.

Cover-Uncover Test for Detecting the Presence of a Latent Squint or Hetereophoria.

The patient is asked to fix a distant spot of light at 6 metres. The right eye is covered and the patient keeps looking to the distant spot of light with his left eye for a few seconds (Fig. 5.5). The cover is removed quickly and the examiner notices if there is any movement in or out, up and down in his covered eye (right eye). This examination is repeated with right eye fixing the spot of light and the left eye put under cover. On removal of the cover the left eye is observed for any

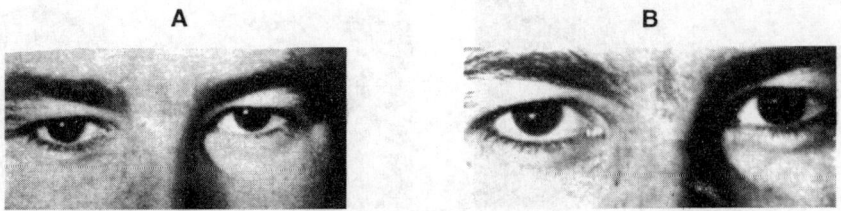

Fig. 5.5: *Photograph taken immediately after uncovering the right eye (**B**). While photograph* **A** *indicates normal forward gaze,* **B** *shows the right eye under cover deviated upwards, a latent deviation which immediately corrects itself to come back photograph* **A**.

deviation. The presence of the deviation in left eye under cover indicates a latent squint. Movement inwards indicates a latent divergent squint, outward indicates a latent convergent squint, a movement upwards under cover indicates hyperphoria and a movement downwards indicates hyperphoria.

It is to be understood that this movement under cover is indicative of recovery movement, that is, movement to regain binocular fixation and therefore, the eye which is not covered will not alter its visual direction as happens in a case of manifest squint.

This cover-uncover test has to be repeated for near fixation distance also. The cover test may also reveal the presence of a latent nystagmus.

In some cases it may become apparent that a child or sometimes an adult who has been referred to an eye surgeon as having ocular deviation or squint, may not be found to have squint on cover/uncover test. He may be a case of psuedo-squint or apparent squint. Such cases may be due to:

1. The presence of a pronounced epicanthic fold on the side of the nose covering the medial canthus partly. This may give the impression of an apparent convergent squint specially when the eyes are looking straight ahead (Fig. 5.6).
2. Undue narrowing of the lateral canthus by reducing the space on the temporal side of the eyeball may cause an impression of a divergent strabismus (Fig. 5.7).
3. In cases of oxycephaly with the reduction of the space in the orbits, the eyeballs look divergent.
4. Presence of a large angle alpha: A large positive (or nasal) angle alpha may produce an apparent divergent strabismus, whereas, the presence of a large negative (temporal) angle alpha may produce an apparent convergent squint.

A little deviation at this stage to show the various "axial" angles of the eye would not be out of place. On would refer to the figures below as given by Lyle and Wybar[13] (Fig. 5.8).

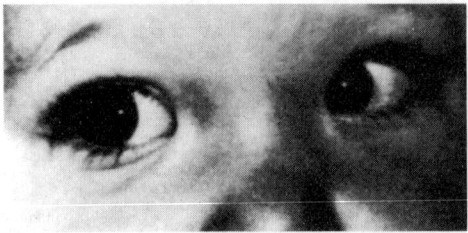

Fig. 5.6: *A case of epicanthus giving the impression of a convergent squint.*

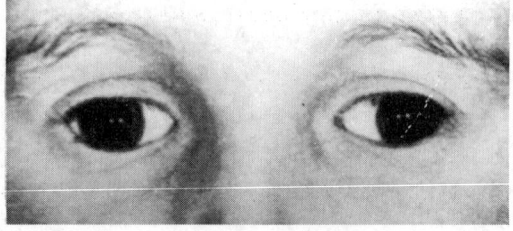

Fig. 5.7: *Narrowing of the palpebral aperture laterally giving the impression of a divergent squint.*

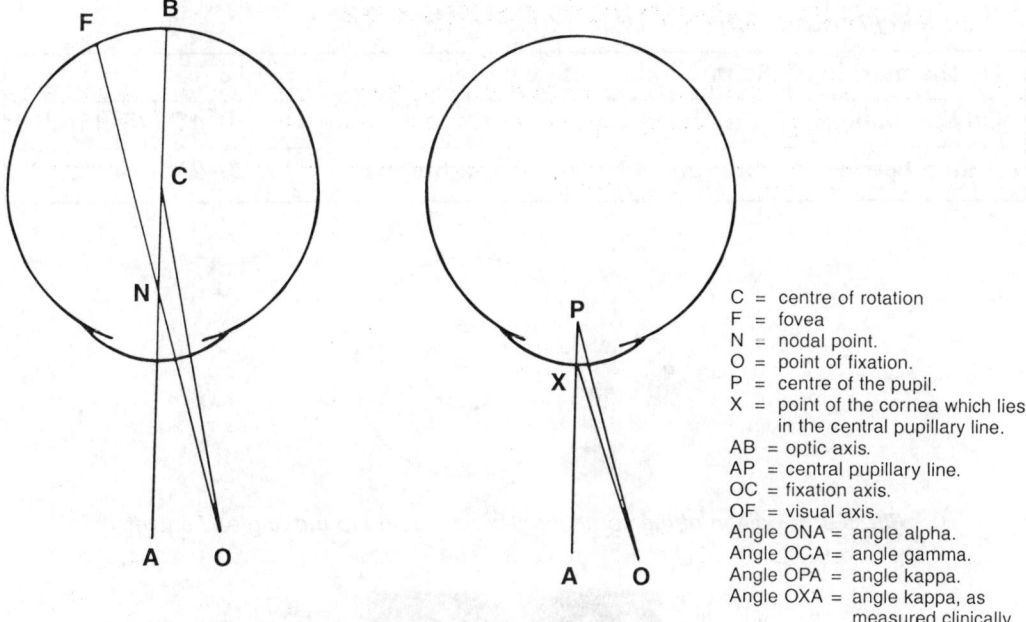

C = centre of rotation
F = fovea
N = nodal point.
O = point of fixation.
P = centre of the pupil.
X = point of the cornea which lies
      in the central pupillary line.
AB = optic axis.
AP = central pupillary line.
OC = fixation axis.
OF = visual axis.
Angle ONA = angle alpha.
Angle OCA = angle gamma.
Angle OPA = angle kappa.
Angle OXA = angle kappa, as
                  measured clinically.

Fig. 5.8: *Various axial angles of the eye.*

It would appear that for practical purposes angle alpha and angle kappa may be treated as equivalent. Further, it is easier to measure angle kappa. This needs emphasising for what Lyle and Wybar[13] say as a large angle alpha is described as a large angle kappa (Von Noorden).

Angle of Deviation

After having been satisfied that one is dealing with a case of true concomitant strabismus, the next part of the examination is to measure the angle of deviation.

Clinically the following common methods are in use.

The Hirschberg Method

It is a simple and at the same time useful and practical method of knowing the amount (angle) of deviation specially in young infants and children.

A torch, or better a torch which makes noise while it lights, is the only instrument needed. The observer sitting directly in front of the child holds a torch light half a metre in front of the patients face. The child is asked to look directly into the light. A corneal reflection of the light is seen in both the eyes. This reflection is in the centre of the pupil in both the eyes, which is normal. If the corneal reflection is seen on the nasal side of the pupil in one eye while it is in the centre of the pupil in the other eye, the deviation is divergent. When this reflection is seen in the temporal side of the pupil the deviation is convergent. And the amount of angle deviation could be obtained roughly as follows:

Position of corneal reflection (Fig. 5.9).

On the margin of the pupil-angle of deviation	12–15°
On the limbus	40–45°(35–45°)
And in between the margin of the pupil and limbus	20–25° (Fig. 5.10).

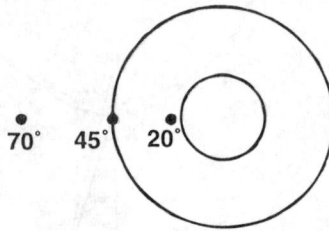

70°   45°   20°

Fig. 5.9: *Position of the corneal reflex as a guide to the angle of squint.*

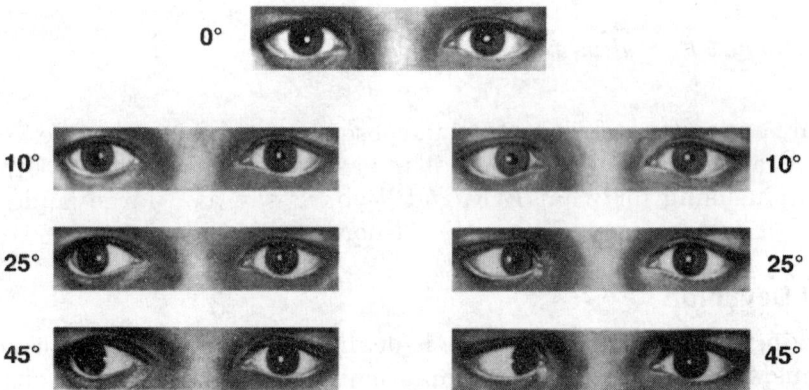

0°

10°   10°

25°   25°

45°   45°

Fig. 5.10: *Photograph showing position of the corneal reflex as a guide to the angle of squint (deviation).*

Corneal Reflection Principle

The same corneal reflection principle could be used using a retinoscopy mirror in a dark room to measure the degree of deviation. Use of priestly Smith tape and measurement of the deviation on the perimeter are now no more used. Instead a prism bar is used along with cover and uncover test to measure the deviation (Fig. 5.11). This method is very useful in the outpatient setting.

Prism-bar and Cover/Uncover Test

Using a prism-bar is more helpful. A prism bar consists of a row of prisms of increasing power. The patient sits in front of a fixation light kept at 6 metres

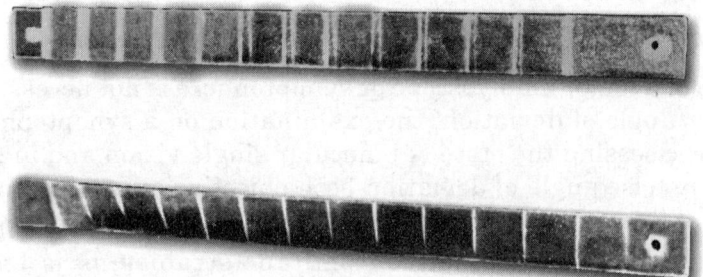

Fig. 5.11: *Photograph showing prism bar, vertical and horizontal.*

and then at 1/3 metre distance. He is asked to look at the fixation light with the right eye while the left eye is covered for a few seconds. Then the cover is moved quickly from the left eye to the right eye and the deviation of the left eye—inwards, outwards, upwards or downwards is noticed.

When the left eye moves inwards to take up fixation—a prism base in is placed before the left eye and the cover test repeated to see whether the deviation of the left eye behind the prism bar (bar in place) is neutralised. The prism bar is moved up and down till the deviation of the left eye is fully neutralised. This gives the strength of the base in prism (in prism dioptre) as the angle (amount) of deviation of the left eye.

With the left eye deviating outwards, the prism bar with base out prism is placed in front of the left eye. And similarly one can know the vertical deviation by placing the prism bar with prism base up and down before the deviating left eye as the case may be. The procedure is repeated a few times so that the angle of deviation is fairly and accurately assessed. The procedure is repeated covering right eye and keeping the left eye open and measuring the deviation of right eye in the same way as that of the left eye just described. While performing the prism bar and cover test, both for distance and near, these should be assessed with the patient first wearing his correction glass and then with the glasses off or removed.

Analysis of these four figures: This *would allow* evidence about the part played by accommodation in the amount of the deviation. Thus, the amount of deviation for distance fixation with the glass (with full correction) excludes accommodation. This gives an idea of the basic or static angle of squint. If the correction of the refractive error is inadequate, accommodation is uncontrolled and one obtains a variable angle of squint (called the dynamic deviation or the dynamic angle of squint).

While using prism bar, two (a pair) are necessary, one for measuring the horizontal deviation and the other for the vertical deviation. In cases of eccentric-fixation or where the deviating eye is blind, prism and cover test cannot be performed.

b. Examination of the Angle of Deviation on a Synoptophore

While the use of a major amblyoscope or synoptophore is not necessary to assess the amount or angle of deviation, the examination on a synoptophore helps in finding out or assessing the state of binocular single vision and in so doing one also gets the precise angle of deviation both objective and subjective.

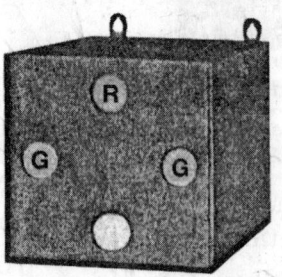

Fig. 5.12 a: Worth's four-dot test.

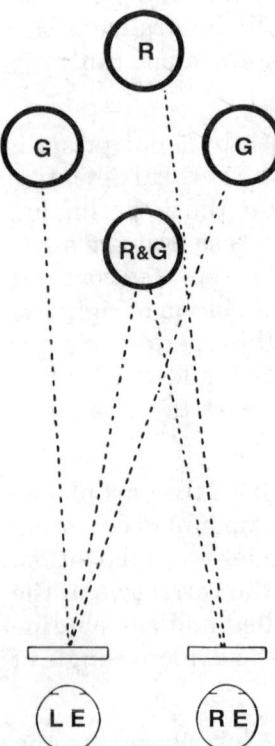

Fig. 5.12 b: Worth's four-light test. R indicates red and G indicates green.

The next stage and an important one in examining cases of concomitant strabismus is to assess the presence and state of binocular single vision.

This could be done using a synoptophore or in an OPD setting using a worth four-dot light test (Fig. 5.12 A and 15.12 B).

Worth's four-light test: It is useful for confirming the presence of binocular single vision and for ascertaining the dominant eye. The apparatus consists of a box containing four plates of glass arranged in diamond formation which are illuminated internally. The two lateral plates of glass are green, the upper one is red and the lower one is white. The patient wears a red and green glass, red glass in front of right eye and the green one in front of the left. The patient is seated 5 to 6 metres away from the light.

i.   A patient with binocular single vision, will see four lights—red above, two green laterally and one pink/white below.

ii. A convergent squinting case with binocular vision will see five lights, three green and two red (Fig. 5.13).

iii. When he is suppressing with the squinting eye, he would see two red lights (left eye suppressing) or three green lights — right eye suppressing (Figs. 5.14 and 5.15).

iv. When he is alternating, he would see 2 or 3 lights alternatively.

While with Worth's four-light test one is able to find out if the subject has binocular single vision, its grade (as mentioned above) can only be examined using a major synoptophore.

Use of Synoptophore

With this instrument an orthoptist gets the following informations.

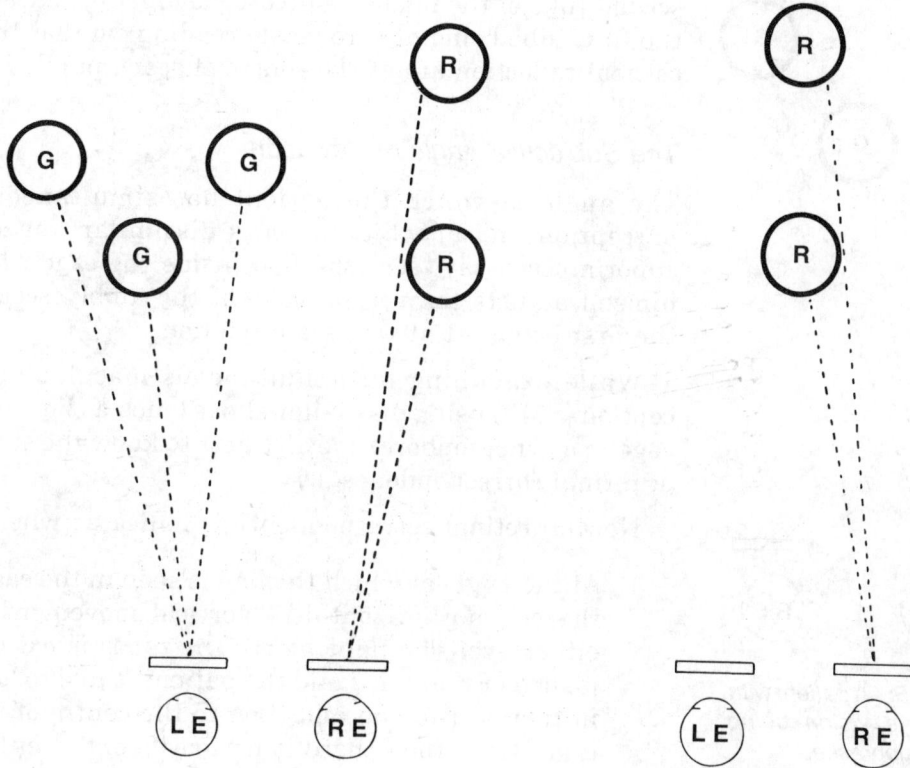

Fig. 5.13: *A patient with convergent squint and binocular vision.*

Fig. 5.14: *A patient with left eye vision being suppressed.*

a. A measurement of the angle of deviation.

b. The state of binocular single vision, which has the following three components or grades:

   i. Simultaneous perception — simultaneous macular or foveal perception;

  ii. Fusion and its range (amplitude); and

 iii. Stereopsis or stereoscopic vision.

The Objective Angle of Deviation

The angle of deviation is estimated on a major amblyoscope/synoptophore. In this instrument one tube projects the picture of a lion (say before the left eye) and the other tube projects the picture of a cage placed before the right eye.

The examination begins by finding the angle at which the tubes of the instrument must be placed so that when the patient is asked to fix the test object, first with one eye and then with the other, there is no corrective movement of the second eye (when it takes up fixation) or by finding the angle at which the

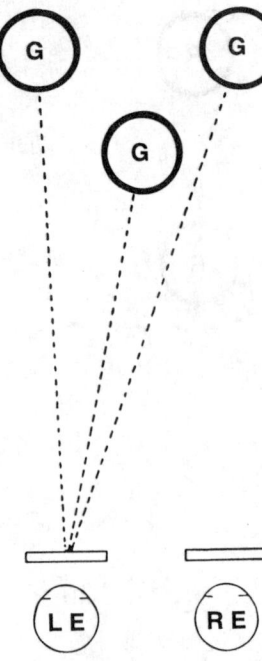

Fig. 5.15: *A patient with right eye vision being suppressed.*

second tube of the major amblyoscope must be placed, the first tube being at zero (scale reading) so that the corneal reflection are at the centre of seach pupil.

The Subjective Angle of Deviation

The angle at which the patient has simultaneous perception and at which he sees dissimilar images superimposed say "sees the lion inside the cage". He himself adjusts the second tube of the amblyoscope, the first being set at zero scale-reading.

While examining for simultaneous macular perception (SMP) using dissimilar slides (such as lion and cage in a synoptophore) one also gets to know the state of retinal correspondence, etc.

Normal retinal correspondence is indicated when

1. At the angle at which the lion is seen in the cage, there is no horizontal or vertical movement of either eye. The light before the tubes is extinguished or reapplied and the patient is told to look in turn at the lion and then to the centre of the cage. Even then there is no movement of either eye.

2. The reflection from the tubes upon the cornea are symmetrically disposed and their position remains unchanged during the test.

3. The scale reading of subjective angle of deviation corresponds with the recorded objective angle.

These clinical findings indicate that the patient has achieved superimposition of images in space by moving the pictures so that these images are focussed simultaneously one on each fovea.

Any of these three indicates that there is normal retinal corresponds or that the image in the two eyes are focussed on corresponding retinal points (the two fovea).

When the patient attempts superimposition of the images (lion and cage as described above), but one image always disappears at the objective angle of deviation and reappears immediately at the other side (when the tube is carried past the objective angle) indicates that basically the sensorial relationship between the two eyes is normal, but is marked by central suppression.

Abnormal retinal correspondence (ARC) with lion and cage in the two arms of the synoptophore as described above is indicated in the following.

1. When at the angle at which the lion is seen in the cage, one or the other eye has to make a movement in order to take up central fixation. Extinguishing the light in front of each eye in turn and asking the patient to look at the centre of each picture makes its obvious.

2. The corneal reflection (from the tube upon the cornea) are asymmetrically placed on the cornea. The reflection in the fixing eye is centrally located (while the eye is fixing) while in the deviating eye, it is temporal or nasal to the centre depending whether it is a divergent or convergent eye.

3. The scale reading at the point of superimposition, the subjective angle is different from the objective angle.

4. At the objective angle, both pictures are seen simultaneously but instead of being seen as superimposed they appear to be situated in two different directions.

Fusion

The second grade of binocular vision is fusion or true fusion with some amplitude. The strength of fusion or its range lies in the ability to converge and diverge to the maximum extent keeping the similar pictures superimposed in a synoptophore. With convergence, fusion can and should be maintained for at least 25° of convergence, whereas fusion cannot be maintained beyond 4° to 6° of divergence.

So far vertical range of fusion is concerned, it varies between 2 Δ to 4 Δ prism dioptre. In practice, it is estimated very rarely except when a vertical deviation is present. Similarly torsional range of fusion is rarely estimated and it varies from 6° to 10°.

Stereoscopic Vision or Depth Perception

A large selection of slides is available for judging stereoscopic vision as also the amplitude of fusion as these are the basic pillars of binocular single vision (a defect of which may cause diplopia). A pair of similar pictures with different controls such as the rabbits or the mouse is used for this (fusion) perception.

REFERENCES

1. Brown, H. W.: The cover-test, in Allen, J. H. (Ed.) *Strabismus Ophthalmic Symposium*. St. Louis, CV Mosby Company, 1958. p. 225.
2. Brown E. V. L.: Net average Yearly change in refraction of atropinised eyes from birth to beyond middle age. *Arch. Ophthalmol.* 19: 719, 1938.
3. Burian, H. M.: Normal and anomalous correspondence, in Allen J. H. (Ed.) *Strabismus Ophthalmic Symposium*. St. Louis, C. V. Mosby Company, p. 184, 1958.

4. Chavasse, F. B.: *Worth's Squint or the Binocular Reflexes and the Treatment of Strabismus.* Philadelphia, P. Blackiston's Son & Co, 1939.

5. Duke Elder, S.: *System of Ophthalmology*, Vol. 3, Part 2 *Congenital deformities*, London, Henry Kimpton, 1964.

6. Guyton, D. L.: Remote optical systems for ophthalmic examinations. *Trans Am. Ophthalmol. Soc.*, 89: 869, 1986.

7. Hardesty, H. H.: Diagnosis of paretic vertical rotators. *Am. J. Ophthalmol.*, 56: 818, 1963.

8. Helveston E. M.: Two-step for diagnosing paresis of vertically acting extraocular muscle. *Am. J. Ophthalmol.* 64 : 914, 1967.

9. Ingram, R. M. and Barr, A.: Refraction of one-year old children after cycloplegia with Cyclopentolate: Comparison with findings after atropinisation. *Brit. J. Ophthalmol.*, 63: 340, 1979.

10. Jacobson, S. G., Mohindra, I. and Held R.: Visual acuity of infants with ocular diseases. *Am. J. Ophthalmol.*, 93 : 198, 1982.

11. Kiff, A. D. and Lepard, C.: Visual responses in premature infants use of optokinetic nystagmus to estimate visual development. *Arch. Ophthalmol.*, 75 : 631, 1966.

12. Lepard, C. W.: Comparative changes in the error of refraction between fixing and amblyopic eyes during growth and development. *Am.J. Ophthalmol.*, 80 : 483, 1975.

13. Lyle T. K. and Wybar K. C.: Lyle and Jackson's - *Practical Orthoptics in the Treatment of Squint,* 5th edn. London, H. K. Lewis and company Ltd, 1967.

14. Noorden, G. K. Von and Olson, C. L.: Diagnosis and surgical management of vertically incomitant horizontal strabismus. *Am. J. Ophthalmol.*, 60 : 23, 1965.

15. Noorden, G. K. Von and Crawford M. L. J.: The sensitive period. *Trans Ophth. Soc. U. K.,* 99: 442, 1980.

16. Parks, M. M.: Isolated cyclovertical muscle palsy. *Arch ophthalmol.*, 60: 1022, 1958.

17. Romano, P. E. and Noorden, G. K. Von: Limitations of cover test in detecting Strabismus. *Am. J. Ophthalmol.*, 77 : 10, 1971.

18. Roper, K. N. and Bannon, R. E.: Diagnostic values of monocular occlusion. *Arch. Ophthalmol.*, 31 : 316, 1944.

19. Scobee, R. G.: *The Oculorotatory Muscles,* 2nd edn. St. Louis, C. V. Mosby Co., 1952.

20. Sloane, A. E.: Analysis of methods of measuring diplopia fields' - Introduction of device for such measurements. *Arch. Ophthalmol.*, 46 : 277, 1951.

21. Slataper, F. J.: Age norms of refraction and vision. *Arch. Ophthalmol.*, 43 : 466, 1950.

22. Spielman, A.: A translucent occulder for study eye positions under unilateral or bilateral covertest. *Am. Orthopt.*, J. 36 : 65, 1986.

23. Toosi, S. H. and Noorden G. K. Von: Effect of isolated inferior oblique muscle myectomy in the management of Superior oblique muscle palsy. *Am. J. Ophthalmol.*, 88: 602, 1979.

24. Urist, M. J.: Head tilt in vertical muscle palsy. *Am. J. Ophthalmol.* 69: 1970.

25. Urist, M. J.: Psuedostrabismus caused by abnormal configuration of eyelid margins. *Am. J. Ophthalmol.*, 75 : 455, 1973.

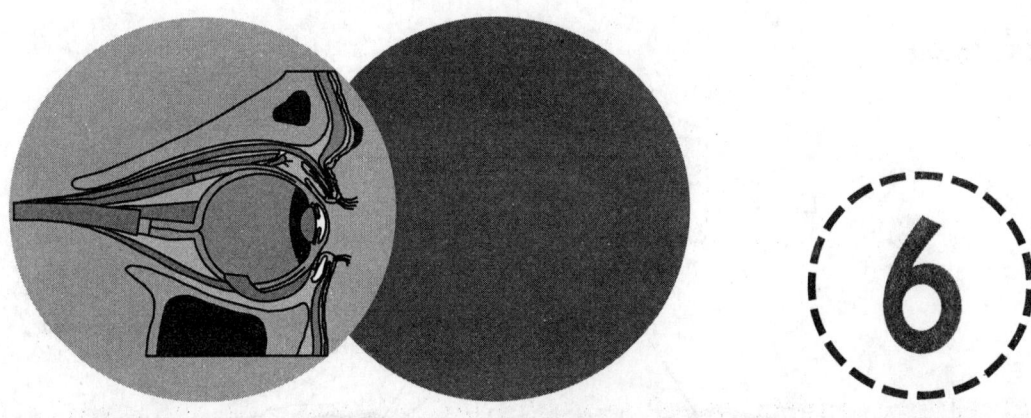

6

Sensory Adaptation in Concomitant Squints Including Amblyopia

The presence of a manifest squint or deviation causes confusion and diplopia. Different objects are imaged on corresponding retinal points in the two eyes (the two fovea) and, are therefore, seen in the same visual direction and overlap. This causes confusion (Fig. 6.1).

On the other hand when one and the same object is imaged in the two eyes on disparate or non-corresponding retinal areas (fovea of the fixing eye and a point in peripheral retina of the deviating eye), they (images) are seen in different visual directions, that is, these are seen as two which is diplopia. Two images of the same object arise together into consciousness with the result that a second similar image is seem to one side of the fixation point. This is diplopia (Fig. 6.2).

Confusion is often not reported voluntarily but when patients do notice overlap of the different foveal images, they find it very distressing. On the other hand, diplopia is a common complaint. This occurs in every patient who has adequate vision in each eye and in whom an acute relative deviation of the visual axis has developed.

To avoid these, confusion and diplopia, the visual system has at its disposal two mechanism-suppression and development of anomalous retinal correspondence. And closely related to suppression is another mechanism-that is amblyopia wherein, the vision in the deviating eye is reduced. These three help the patient to gain comfortable single monocular vision or an anomalous

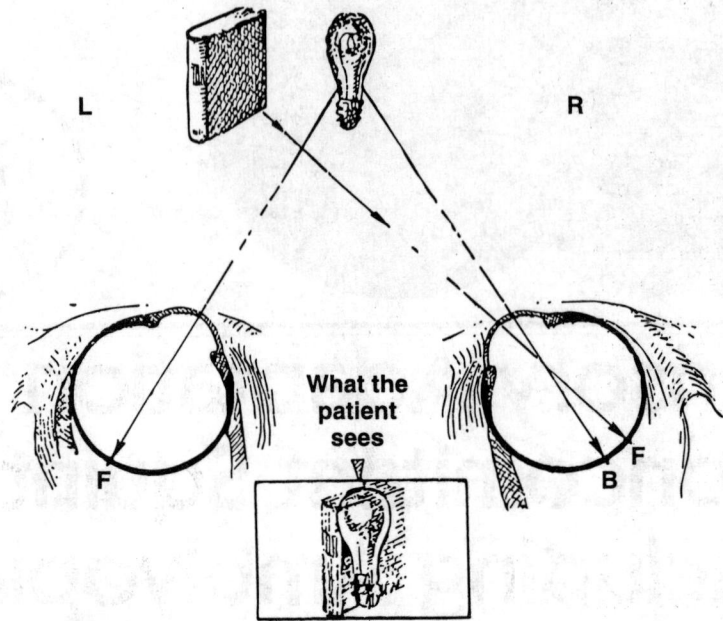

Fig. 6.1: *Light being viewed by the fovea F of the left eye and the fovea of the right esotropic eye views the book. The patient sees the book and light superimposed. Both images are interpreted as in straight ahead position—the visual direction of the fovea. This is confusion.*

form of binocular single vision. These, thus, constitute nature's way of adapting to the altered situation caused by deviation of one eye uniocularly or alternately.

DIPLOPIA

In a convergent squint, the fixation object is viewed by the fovea of the non-squinting or normal eye, while in the deviating eye its image is formed on a point in the peripheral retina, nasal to the fovea. This results in cerebral impression of a false object situated on the temporal side of the true object. This is a homonymous diplopia or uncrossed diplopia (Figs 6.2 and 6.3). The angle between the line of projection of the stimulated retinal point of the squinting eye and the assumed line of projection of the fovea of the non squinting eye is the angle of squint (deviation).

In a divergent squint: the fixation object is viewed by the fovea of the normal (or non-squinting eye) and by a peripheral retinal point situated on the temporal side of the fovea of the squinting eye. This later point being situated in a part of the retina, which normally receives stimuli from objects in the nasal part of the visual field, cerebral impression of a second object situated on the nasal side of the true object. This gives a crossed or heteronymous diplopia (Fig. 6.4). True image is the image of the non-squinting normal eye and false image is the image of the squinting eye.

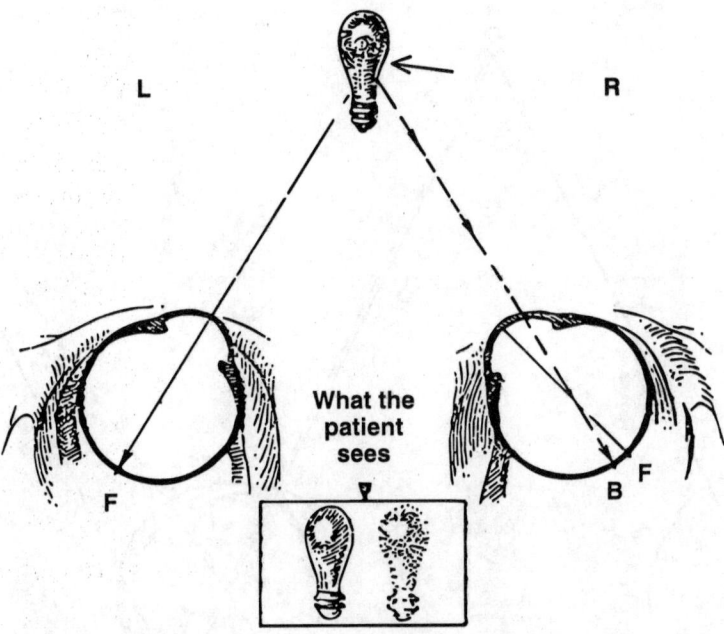

Fig. 6.2: *A patient with right eye esotropia. The light is imaged on the fovea F of the fixing left eye and on point B nasal to the fovea of the right esotropic eye. The patient sees two lights (diplopia). As point B is nasal to fovea F the second light is seen to the light—homonymous or uncrossed diplopia.*

Diplopia is binocular, that is both eyes (the fixing eye and the deviating squinting) have to do seeing to cause diplopia. But a different type of diplopia also exists, the uniocular diplopia which has nothing to do with concomitant squint cases (except occasionally during treatment of strabismic-amblyopia).

Monocular diplopia is sometimes complained of in cases of incipient cataract because of different refractive indices of the lens layers in such eyes. Actually this is polyopia where the moon may appear two or three instead of the normal one.

Suppression

One of the means by which double vision and confusion could be avoided or overcome is suppression. The image of an object formed on the retina of the squinting eye is not perceived but is mentally ignored or neglected partly or completely. The process of suppression is the result of a cerebral inhibition. This gives the fovea of the normal (non-squinting) eye complete dominance so that it forms the centre of attention and the patient adjusts himself to the environment by means of a uniocular type of perception There is an active inhibition of the image from the squinting eye in the cerebral centres and as

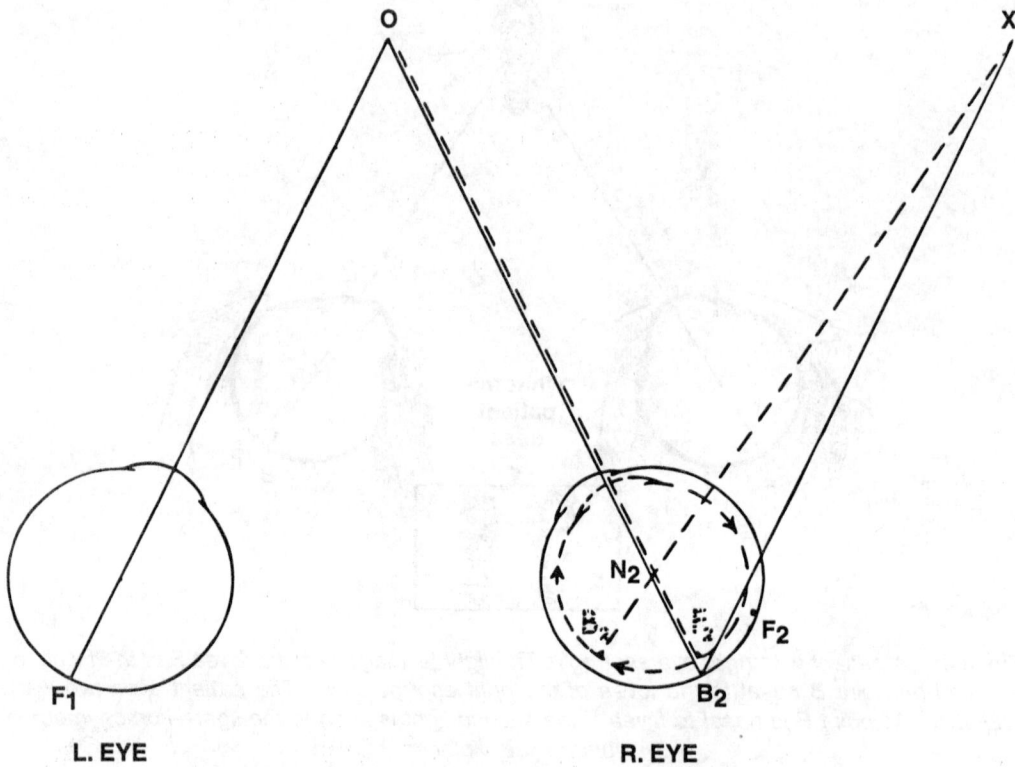

Fig. 6.3: *Homonymous diplopia in a right convergent squint.*

such, the visual acuity of this eye suffers causing more or less a perceptual blindness.

Such a suppression has two phases or is of two types:

(a) Facultative, and
(b) Obligatory inhibition.

Facultative type of inhibition In this type, suppression of the image from the squinting eye occurs so long the eye is deviating. The moment this eye takes up fixation, the inhibition of the image (or visual impression) of the eye disappears and there is an immediate return to the more or less normal visual function. This is typically seen in alternating squint cases where suppression is transferred immediately from one eye to the other on changing fixation. In this way each eye retains good visual function (Fig. 6.5).

Obligatory inhibition So long a squinting eye is deviating, there is suppression from this eye. Even when the squinting eye is forced to take up fixation because of better visual acuity the suppression persists.

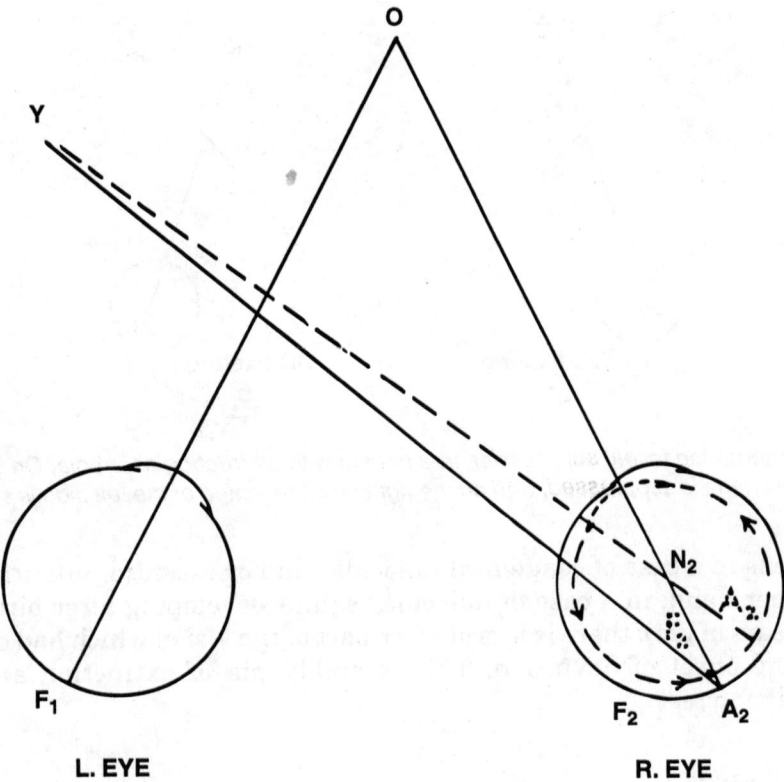

Fig. 6.4: *Heteronymous diplopia in a right divergent squint.*

It is typically seen in a case of uniocular convergent squint where the non-deviating normal eye is chosen for fixation (because it has a better visual acuity) and the squinting deviating eye continues to have suppression which in due course becomes obligatory and fixed.

In the early stages of the development of a uniocular squint, the inhibition is facultative and as time goes on and there is no treatment to correct the deviation – the inhibition becomes obligatory with the suppression of the image this eye at cortical level. This in turn leads to consequential dimunition of the visual function and visual acuity of the deviating eye.

In a young child when the binocular reflexes are still in a state of flux, there is a rapid transition from the facultative to the obligatory stage of inhibition. But in an older child (where these reflexes have become well-established) this is not feasible and the obligatory inhibition may persists.

If a child is born with squint or he develops the deviation in the early months after birth, the presence of deviation precludes the development or further development of central vision. This failing of vision is amblyopia of arrest. And

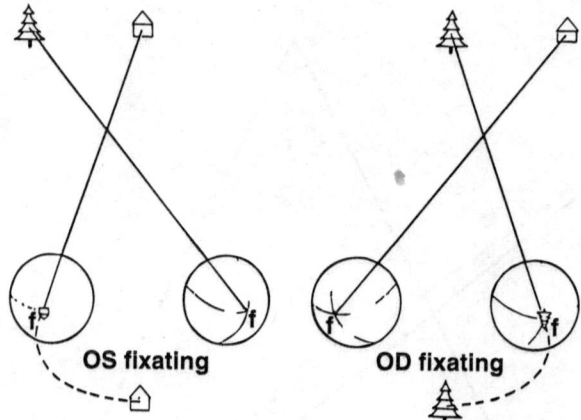

Fig. 6.5: *Alternating foveal suppression in a patient with alternating esotropia. On the left side the right eye image is suppressed, and on the right side the image of the left side is suppressed.*

this happens in a case of congenital uniocular and or essential infantile squint. On the other hand, in a case of uniocular squint developing after birth (in the first few years of life), there is loss of all or part of the vision which had developed prior to the onset of deviation. This is amblyopia of extinction along with amblyopia of arrest.

Eccentric-Fixation

Following obligatory inhibition, the fixation of the squinting eye may suffer. A non-foveal-retinal receptor (in the squinting eye) assumes a foveal or straight-ahead form of projection. This therefore, becomes the point of reference around which the other retinal receptors are ranged as a result of a change in the spatial projection of all the receptors. This eccentric retinal point has been termed as a false-macula or false-fovea and has less of visual acuity value. It is an uniocular and not a binocular condition.

When in a squinting eye abnormal retinal correspondence (ARC) (being discussed later in this chapter also), develops a point in the squinting eye other than the fovea takes up fixation as an adaptation to produce binocular single vision (BSV). This is pseudo-fovea. This point is, however, flexible for the squinting eye can still have foveal fixation when it is fixing or made to fix straight ahead. In such cases of unconsolidated ARC, the abnormal correspondence exists only when the two eyes are used together and disappears immediately on covering either the squinting or non-squinting eye.

In some cases of ARC, however, the abnormal state remains in the squinting eye despite the covering of the non squinting eye so that there is an obligatory or permanent type of perversion of the projection. In these cases the ARC is associated with an eccentric or non-central fixation.

Mapping Suppression Scotoma

The extent of suppression scotoma can be clinically estimated by the use of prisms. By placing prisms of increasing strength in front of the eye with suppression scotoma, one would soon find a prism with which the patient experiences diplopia. While the normal eye continues seeing a small fixation light, its image in the squinting deviating eye is now thrown out of the region of the suppression scotoma onto a retinal area that is not suppressed. The dioptric power and direction of the base of the prism required to produce diplopia is a measure of the extent of suppression scotoma.

Abnormal (or Anomalous) Retinal Correspondence

Another sensory adaptation of a squinting eye is the development of abnormal retinal correspondence (ARC) as shown in Fig. 6.6. It is an abnormality of binocular visual function which occurs in some cases of concomitant squint as an adaptation to the ocular deviation in an attempt to avoid diplopia and confusion. Chavasse (1939) wrote "The first sign of ARC is the ability to project correctly inspite of deviation of one eye in relation to the body in space). It is an attempt to restore some semblance of binocular vision".

In consists of a re-arrangement of the common visual direction of the retinal elements of the two eyes, as corresponding retinal elements loose their common visual direction (Burian[9], 1951).

It is not caused by nor is associated with any anatomical retinal anomaly but is essentially a functional adaptation of cortical origin in which eventually not only the fovea of the fixing eye becomes associated binocularly with a point on the retina other than the fovea of the squinting eye, but also the entire retina of the two eyes become functionally linked in an abnormal binocular association.

Anomalous correspondence is an attempt by the patient to recover/regain binocular co-operation when the visual axes are misaligned. To a degree this attempt is successful. The anomalous binocular vision that develops is a functional state superior to that prevailing in the presence of suppression in alternating strabismus.

The visual input from a suppressed area is limited and is of no apparent benefit to binocular vision other than elimination of diplopia and confusion. The question of how often ARC is encountered in untreated cases of concomitant squint cannot be answered unequivocally. Its rate of occurrence is high in infantile esotropia, less common in exotropia and uncommon in vertical strabismus.[32]

Anomalous correspondence presumably adapts the sensory visual system to the abnormal motor condition created by the deviation in an effort to restore some semblance of binocular co-operation. If the fovea of the fixing eye acquires a common visual direction with an area in the retina of the deviated eye on

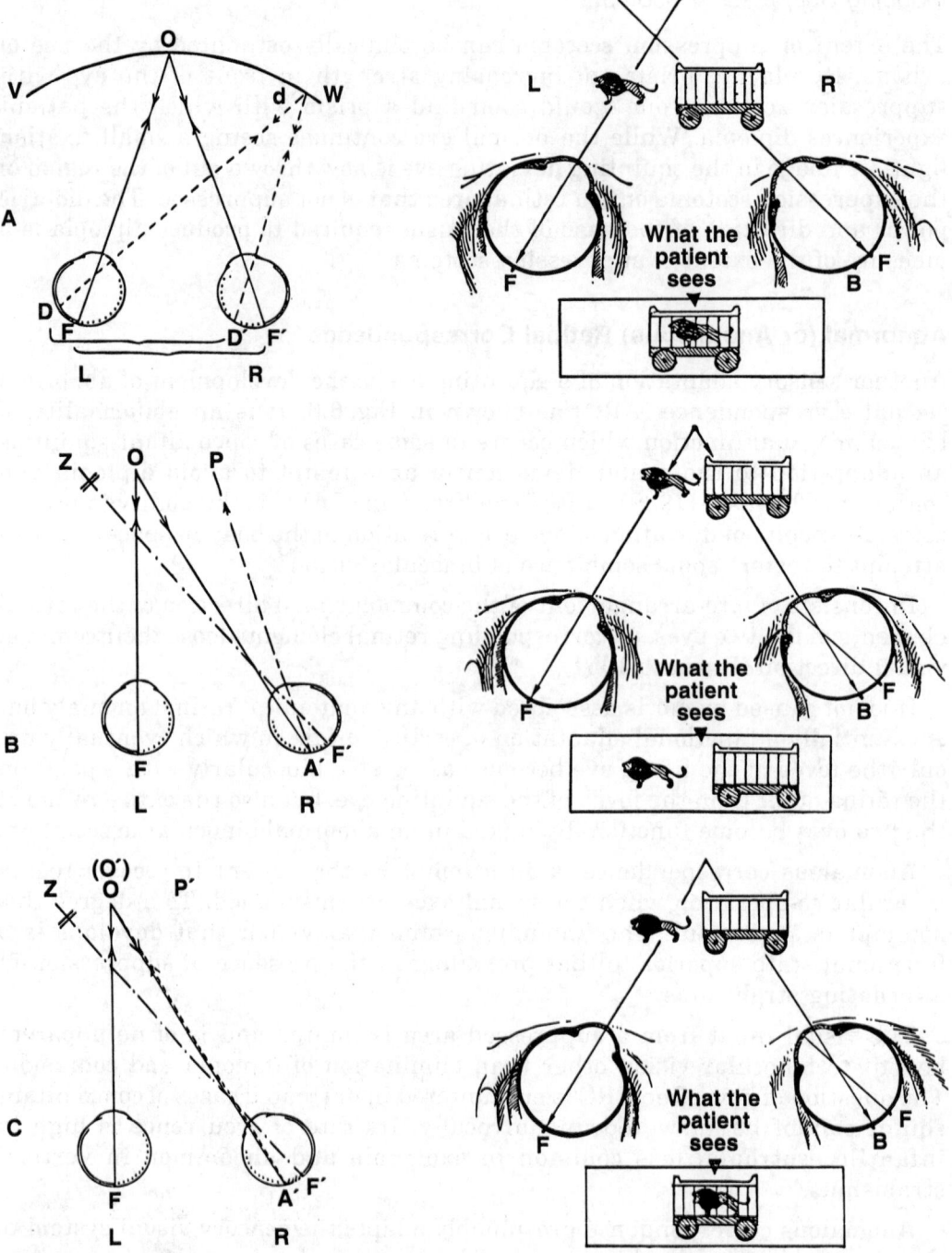

Fig. 6.6: *Retinal correspondence illustrated.* **A** *Normal retinal correspondence.* **B** *Normal retinal correspondence in a case of right convergent squint.* **C** *Abnormal retinal correspondence in a case of right convergent squint (harmonious).*

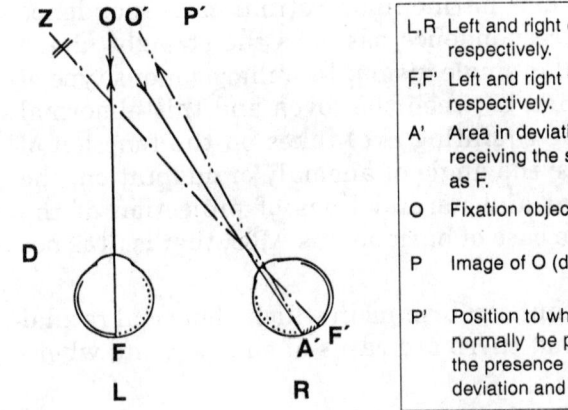

L,R	Left and right eyes, respectively.	O'	Projection of O in unharmonious abnormal retinal correspondence.
F,F'	Left and right foveae, respectively.	O"	Projection of O in harmonious abnormal retinal correspondence.
A'	Area in deviating right eye receiving the same image as F.	Z	Direction of deviation of right eye
O	Fixation object.	d	Object situated to the right side of the fixation object on the horopter.
P	Image of O (diplopia)	D, D'	Corresponding points in orthophoria.
P'	Position to which O would normally be projected in the presence of a manifest deviation and NRC.	VW	Horopter

Fig. 6.6: **D** *Abnormal retinal correspondence in a case of right convergent squint (unharmonious).*

which the fixation point or object is imaged, the deviation is fully neutralised sensorially, that is, the shift in the visual direction has fully offset the amount of deviation. In this situation the sensory adaptation is more successful and one speaks of harmonious ARC when both images in the red-filter test coincide. If the amount of the shift in visual directions does not fully compensate for the deviation, the adaptation is not complete and one speaks of unharmonious ARC.

Abnormal Retinal correspondence is of two types:

1. Harmonious ARC, and
2. Unharmonious.

Harmonious Type of ARC

Normally in a squinting eye the image of the object of fixation falls on a point nasal or temporal to the fovea depending on the type of squint convergent and divergent.

When in such a squinting eye, abnormal retinal correspondence develops of the type harmonious (Fig. 6.6 C), the image of the object of fixation is appreciated by the deviating eye in a straight ahead (or foveal) direction. The angle, thus, formed between the abnormal and normal lines of projection of the squinting eye is termed the "Angle of anomaly" or the angle of adaptation. This angle of anomaly in the harmonious type of ARC is equal to the angle of squint.

Unharmonious Abnormal Retinal Correspondence

Normally a fixation object is viewed or appreciated by the fovea of the normal eye and by a point other than the fovea (on nasal side to it in convergent squint) of the squinting convergent eye. When harmonious retinal correspondence develops, this point of abnormal correspondence assumes the straight ahead (foveal) fixation to give rise to binocular single vision. In unharmonious type of ARC (Fig. 6.6 D), a point on the retina between the fovea and this abnormal point of fixation on the retina (in the squinting eye) takes on the function of straight ahead (foveal) fixation. Thus, the angle of anomaly or adaptation, the angle formed between the abnormal and normal lines of projection of the squinting eye is smaller than that in a case of harmonious ARC, that is, it is not true angle of deviation.

Clinically we have cases of concomitant strabismus in which abnormal retinal correspondence is likely to develop and there are cases of such squints where ARC is unlikely to occur.

Cases in which ARC is Likely to Develop[32]

i. The majority of cases likely to develop ARC are those of concomitant convergent squints of low to moderate degree, the condition being less likely to be found in deviation greater than + 20° to + 25° or 25" to 30" prism dioptre. Suppression is the rule in patient with larger deviations.

ii. Convergent squints of early onset that is, up to the age of three years and infantile esotropia specially when treatment has been neglected. The instability of the binocular reflexes in these cases lead to replacement of normal reflex development by abnormal binocular reflexes.

iii. Abnormal retinal correspondence is common in alternating convergent squints particularly when it is of the congenital or essential type.

iv. It is also common in uniocular squints where the patient has retained the ability to fix easily with the habitually deviating eye.

v. It is also to be found in those with residual postoperative deviation.

Cases of Squint in which ARC is Unlikely to Occur

i. ARC is generally not found in cases of primary divergent squints irrespective of the age. In these cases there is no visual reward from abnormal retinal correspondence. Also in divergent squints many cases are intermittent to start with and by the time the deviation becomes constant, the binocular single visual function has developed.

ii. Convergent squint cases of late onset say after the age of fifteen or sixteen year. In these cases chances are that binocular reflexes have already fully developed and as such they cannot be easily replaced by abnormal reflexes.

iii. Convergent squint cases with deviation greater than + 25° to + 30° or more. In these cases, the image in the deviating eye is formed in the peripheral retina, hence, poorly defined and as such easily suppressed.

iv. Cases of convergent squints of variable angle of deviation — In such cases, no particular area can be established as pseudo-fovea.

Suppression in ARC is a variable feature. In the early stages of development of ARC, there is suppression of the fovea in the deviating eye in order to avoid confusion. There is also suppression of that part of the surrounding retina projection from which may cause diplopia. Subsequently a fresh attempt to obtain some form of 'binocular single vision' occurs and the fovea of the habitually fixing eye begins its association with a new retinal area of the deviating eye, either the psuedo-foveal or the para-foveal area. Thus, a new range of corresponding points develops throughout both retina. Such a positive adaptation avoids the need for the suppression.

Detection of ARC.

A variety of methods and tests have been described for detecting the presence of this binocular anomaly. Of these two are in common practice (a) Examination on major amblyoscope, and (b) After-image test.

Examination on Major Amblyoscope (see Fig. 7.2)

As usual both the objective and subjective measurements are made of the deviation. In objective measurement — using foveal-sized pictures (in the slides) say lion before the left eye (fixing eye) and the cage before the right eye (the deviating eye), the left tube is set at zero on the scale and the right tube (with the deviating eye) is moved till the corneal reflex in this eye appears in the centre of the cornea as in the left eye. At this point both the pictures, the lion and the cage are seen at the same time but not superimposed indicating lack of normal retinal correspondence. This movement of the right tube (deviating eye) gives the objective angle.

In the subjective method, the patient himself moves the tube (in front of the deviating eye) till the corneal reflex for this eye appears in the centre of the cornea and he feels that the lion is well inside the cage.

Angle of Anomaly

The difference between the subjective angle and the objective angle is known as the angle of anomaly or the angle of adaptation. (The objective angle minus the subjective angle is the angle of anomaly). When both the objective and subjective angle are equal, the angle of anomaly is zero and the retinal correspondence is normal.

(1) In harmonious type of ARC: The patient subjectively superimposes the picture at zero, whereas on objective measurement, he shows say an angle of deviation of 20° in the squinting eye. Hence, objective minus subjective angle, that is the angle of anomaly is the same as the objective angle (viz. 20°).

(2) In unharmonious type of ARC: The patient himself superimposes the pictures by the right deviating eye at an angle which is smaller than the objective angle of deviation. As before the tube containing the lion (before left eye) is set at zero on the scale. The angle of anomaly is therefore, less than the objective angle.

The ARC found on examination may be unstable and variable and amenable to treatment or it may be stable and constant and thus difficult to eradicate. (And if on further examination, the patient has a good power and range of fusion, nothing need be done to treat such a case of ARC).

The After-Image-Test

Extensively used by Bielschowsky[4] (1938) is accepted as the best method of ascertaining the sensorial relationship between the two eyes. Demonstrating after-image test could be carried out on a synoptophore using after-image slides, or (ii) in the original method using a cylindrical glass tube one feet in length containing a glowing filament. Around the centre of the tube there is a black band with a fixation spot. The tube is attached to its stand in such a way that it could be rotated from the vertical into the horizontal position. One can also use an electronic flash device. In this way after image will form a perfect cross.

A patient with normal retinal correspondence will see the after-image as a symmetrical cross as depicted in Fig. 6.7 A. The visual impulse has been observed independently by both fovea and since these are corresponding points, the centre of both images coincide.

In ARC the after-image is asymmetrical. The images will be alongside each other in a variety of ways since the foves are no longer corresponding points and do not share the same local signs. The vertical line is on to the left in the esotropic patient and to the right in the exotropic patient (Fig. 6.7 B & C). Children may experience difficulties both in appreciating and in describing the after-image. Then again in a patient with right convergent squint and an associated high hypertropia, the image may not appear as clear as above.

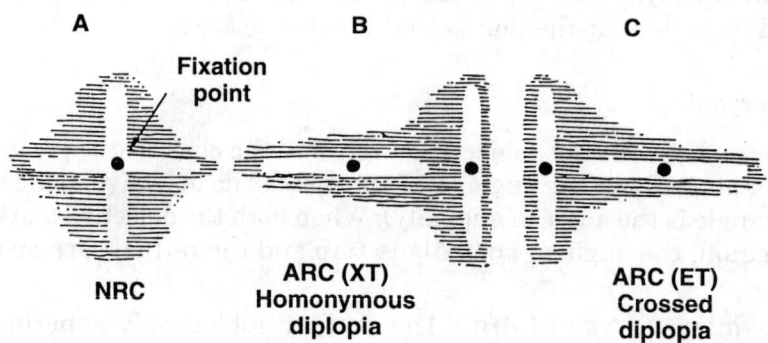

A   **B**   **C**

Fixation point

NRC

ARC (XT)
Homonymous
diplopia

ARC (ET)
Crossed
diplopia

Fig. 6.7: **A** *After–image in an eye with normal retinal correspondence.* **B & C** *After–image in esotropic and exotropic eye.*

Striated Glass Test of Bagolini (1958) Quoted by Noorden[36.]

Striated glass lenses (Fig. 6.8) have been used for demonstrating the presence of ARC. On looking a spotlight or light source through a plain glass with fine striations as in a Maddox Rod, the spot-light appears to be transected by a clear linear streak of light. One such striated glass is put in front of right eye and the other in front of left eye in a trial frame, in a way that the streaks of the two glass appear to be at right angle to each other. With such an arrangement the linear streak of light (of the spotlight) presented to one eye is at right angle to that presented to the other eye. A person with normal binocular-vision or normal retinal correspondence will see the two lines making a cross and bisecting each other at the centre of the spotlight (I). In a patient with manifest deviation and normal retinal correspondence the lines do cross (II) but two light sources are seen and the crossing does not take place at the light source.

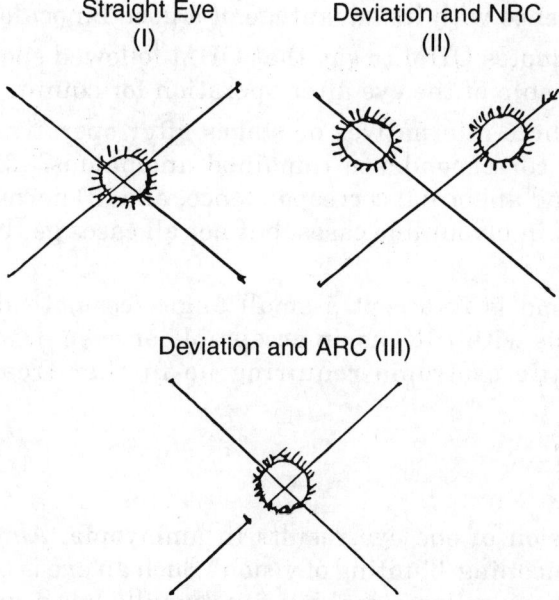

Fig. 6.8: *Bagolini striated–glass test.*

With abnormal retinal correspondence/ARC/ and a deviation, there is a gap in one line because of suppression scotoma where they intersect (III).

Treatment of ARC

It is generally accepted that ARC is a well established adaptation which may follow the development of squint. It is a condition which can become so firmly fixed that eradication is often impossible. A harmonious type of ARC counteracts diplopia and confusion and provides a useful form of binocular vision. Hence, in a large number of cases it is uneconomical to attempt to treat and it is doubtful if the effort is really worthwhile.

In early cases, when ARC is still in the developing state, occlusion of the sound eye may arrest its progress and reduce its stability. Occlusion helps to prevent as well as to cure or lessen the abnormal retinal correspondence. Occlusion is necessary to prevent the continued stimulation of noncorresponding points of the retina in the deviating eye and thus, reduce its stability. In cases of alternating deviation (and where the visual acuity is more or less equal), alternate occlusion should be employed more so in young children. Theoretically, the duration for which occlusion has to be continued is till the time the correct sensorial relationship is re-established. In clinical practice, however, it is a long drawn affair and may not be complied with.

Orthoptic exercises and surgical correction of the deviation do help. But it is doubtful how far these efforts can help a child with ARC to switch back to normal retinal correspondence with its advantage of a good binocular vision.

Von Noorden[36] quotes OHM to say that OHM followed spontaneous changes in sensory relationship of the eye after operation for squint.

He postulates three alternatives or stages after operative correction of the deviation, viz. (1) correspondence remained anomalous, (2) rivalry occurred between normal and abnormal correspondence, and (3) normal correspondence was re-established in favourable cases, but not all cases go through these three stages.

The present trend is to accept a small angle (cosmetically inconspicuous) residual strabismus with ARC as an acceptable or even desirable end stage of therapy in infantile esotropia requiring no further treatment except for amblyopia.

AMBLYOPIA

Habitual suppression of one eye results in amblyopia. *Amplyopia* is derived from Greek word meaning 'blunting of vision'. Such an eye is generally described as one which is structurally normal but functionally has reduced visual acuity. And this reduced visual acuity cannot be fully improved with glasses.

This blunting of vision or poor visual acuity in an eye may be associated with an organic lesion or is without any detectable organic lesion. The latter is pure amblyopia while the former with organic lesion (as for example amblyopia with congenital cataract or that associated with toxic substance) would not be what we mean as functional amblyopia.

Toxic amblyopia is organic amblyopia and outside the scope of the present description. Hence, to avoid confusion, this term should be carefully used.

The condition of functional amblyopia may be explained by a unilateral suppression of foveal-vision and is most of the time unilateral. But one does come across cases of bilateral amblyopia as in cases of high hypermetropia in both eyes in excess of + 7.00 dioptre or associated with astigmatism in excess of + 3 dioptre.

In a number of cases of amblyopia, the reduced visual acuity in the amblyopic eye is associated with deviation (squint) in that eye. Hence, we can divide cases of uniocular amblyopia into sub groups as given in Table 6.1 (Rohatgi[46], 1972).

Table 6.1 **Amblyopia**

Without Squint (Straight eye amblyopia)	With Squint	
	With central fixation	With eccentric fixation
(a) With high hypermetropia in the amblyopic eye anisometropic amblyopia (b) With equal refractive error in both eyes (c) With no significant refractive error	With or without significant refractive error in the amblyopic deviating eye	

Of the two groups, the straight-eye amblyopia group constitutes a large percentage of such cases.

Straight Eye Amblyopia

The first group of straight-eye amblyopia cases have high hypermetropic refractive error in the amblyopic eye. They have been variously called as suppression amblyopia, straight-eye amblyopia and anisometropic amblyopia. Such cases often go unnoticed till the child has a routine school medical examination. The mechanism of such an amblyopia is different from the mechanism in cases of strabismic amblyopia.

Such an amblyopia is obligatory in type but more amenable to treatment than amblyopia in a case of strabismus. A check synoptophore examination may show fair binocular function (simultaneous macular perception, fusion and full stereopsis with little or no suppression) and one can easily rule out eccentric fixation.

If a child is unable to accommodate equally with each eye as happens in anisometropic hypermetropia or if the accommodation does not achieve clear definition as in unilateral astigmatism, the retinal image of the more hypermetropic/astigmatic eye is blurred. This blurred image acts as sensory obstruction to binocular vision and is, therefore, suppressed. This suppression begins when accommodation starts being active that is about the age of 2 to 3 years. The sensitivity to develop suppression and amblyopia gradually decreases till the child reaches 6 to 7 years of age whereafter, visual maturation is complete and the retinocortical pathways and visual centres may become immune to abnormal visual input.

At first, the inhibition is probably facultative and in the nature of a central scotoma but habitual disuse renders it obligatory. Distortion of objects, however, does not occur. In myopia on the other hand, the more myopic eye is used for near work and the less myopic eye for distance vision. Since both the retinas continue to receive adequate stimulation, amblyopia does not develop. In cases of high myopia and more so when one eye is highly myopic (unilateral high myopia) the retina this eye is deprived of adequate vision and clarity and amblyopia may develop in such an eye.

In groups (b) and (c) of straight eye amblyopia -

In these cases either there is no significant refractive error in the eye (as in group c) or both eyes have equal degree of hypermetropia as in (b). To explain why amblyopia does develop in these cases is not easy.

According to Philips (1966) a possible explanation is that, theoretically, a pair of eyes might have very different image-size in spite of being emmetropic or having an equal degree of refractive error. This would occur if two eyes had different axial length with compensatory difference in the cornea and lens to produce equal refraction. And if concentration of rods and cones per unit area is the same in the two eyes, the patient is presented with the problem of anisokonia (different size of the retinal image in the two eyes). The clarity of each image being different makes the problem worse. Depending on the amount of the inequality, the patient may choose to squint or to suppress.

Amblyopia with Squint

Patients who constantly use one eye for fixation as in unilateral squint (and as opposed to alternating fixation pattern in case of alternating squint) are most likely to develop or acquire strabismic amblyopia. Thus, one can expect to find amblyopia more often in esotropes than in exotropes.

In the majority of cases of concomitant squint, specially when one eye has a higher visual acuity, this eye tends to be used in preference to the other. This causes a conditioned inhibition in the neglected deviated eye. This inhibition gradually becomes fixed leading to the development of an obligatory inhibition or amblyopia.

The earlier the age at which inhibition first become operative, the more profound is the amblyopia. Thus, in a case of congenital squint, where the inhibition is present from birth, vision in the squinting deviating eye will remain permanently a little more than the perception of light.

On the other hand, if this inhibition of vision in the squinting eye occurs after the age of 6 or 7 years (when visual maturation is expected to be complete) no such arrest of development or amblyopia is likely to occur. In between, when amblyopia comes up about the age of 3 to 4 years (accommodative convergent squint) recovery of vision is likely to take place upto the level-normal for the age at which inhibition commenced. This was earlier referred to as amblyopia exanopsia (amblyopia of disuse or under stimulation of retina). Such stimulus-deprivation amblyopia is seen in children with opacities of the ocular media — congenital or traumatic cataract, corneal leucoma or following prolonged and indiscriminate patching (occlusion amblyopia). It is not necessary that the anblyopic eye shows deviation or squint.

In addition to the process of developmental arrest (mentioned above) any vision which has not become permanently established and reached the state of an unconditioned fixation reflex, may be actively suppressed (amblyopia of extinction). For, example visual acuity may have developed as far as 6/12 when an obstacle interferes with further normal development.

Further, the visual acuity may after a period of disuse of such an eye may deteriorate to 6/24, this drop is called the amblyopia of extinction. Thus, if a child's eye is bandaged (for a month or so as is done by bandaging the sound eye to help increase VA in the deviating eye) the vision in that eye may drop, to recover again when the obstacle is removed.

The depth of amblyopia and its recovery varies depending, on

a. the degree of VA attained before inhibition became effective,
b. the period during which the extinction of vision remained active, and
c. the age at which amblyopia developed.

Thus, deep amblyopia is a disease of the young children primarily those under the age of four years. Most infants with amblyopia are detected at the age of 2 to 3 years.

On the other hand, when the deviation begins late, say after 7 to 8 years of age, habitual suppression is difficult and amblyopia is less common. An adult with a recent onset of deviation invariably complains of diplopia and the absence of this complaint suggests an earlier onset of the deviation.

Clinical Notes

From clinical point of view, a difference of two lines on a visual acuity chart (Snellen-chart) is commonly used as a diagnostic criteria for amblyopia. However, in a patient with squint in whom the VA in the "amblyopic eye" has improved from 6/36 to 6/12 must still be considered amblyopic while visual acuity in the fixing sound eye is 6/6.

Crowding Phenomenon

In patients with amblyopia, it is always of interest and importance to compare the vision obtained with visual acuity symbols presented in a row to that obtained with isolated symbols like E on a uniform background. According to Von-

Noorden[36, 40], in some patients the difference is quite startling such as when line acuity of 6/36 (-6/30) responds correctly to 6/6 symbols presented singly. This is known as crowding phenomenon.

If standard line acuity is not or cannot be achieved, the probability is high that the vision of the amblyopic eye will regress significantly. Thus, at least, at the completion of treatment, the presence or absence of the crowding phenomenon has significant prognostic value (Von-Noorden, 1990) [36.]

Fixation Pattern of Amblyopic Eye

There are cases of strabisimic amblyopia where the fixation is eccentric rather than being central. These cases of eccentric fixation do not assume central fixation even when the fellow eye is occluded, that is the amblyopic eye remains more or less deviated.

Bangerter's (1953)[14, 15] classification of fixation pattern in amblyopia (Fig. 6.9) is as follows.

1. Central fixation (Foveolar)
2. Eccentric fixation (non-foveolar)   Parafoveal within 2' of the fovea
3. No fixation (erratic) - no definite   Paramacular between 2' to 4'
   area of fixation around the true   away from the true fovea,
   fovea (Peripheral)   Centrocaecal Greater than 4'
                                          between the macula and the
                                          optic disc, paracentral around
                                          the optic disc.

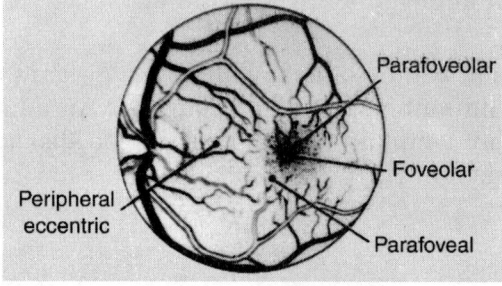

Fig. 6.9: Amblyopia — fixation pattern photograph.

The prevalence of eccentric fixation in strabismic amblyopia has been reported by different authors varying from 23% (Scully, 1961)[47] to 82% (Harada and Hayashi, 1958, quoted from Von-Noorden[36]).

For diagnosing and treating eccentric-fixation, Cuppers of Giessen[32, 36] has devised visuscope, euthyscope and coordinator. Since then space — coordinator and keeler projectoscope have been added to the list which originally began with devising pleotophore, etc. by Bangerter.

Cover Test and Corneal Reflex Method can diagnose only gross degree of eccentric-fixation and thus, many of these cases can remain undiagnosed and wrongly treated in the absence of these diagnostic instruments.

With the help of a visuscope (a modified ophthalmoscope), Cuppers first localised accurately the eccentric fixation.

A number of modern ophthalmoscope have a built-in fixation target that helps in diagnosing the eccentric fixation. Once diagnosed, Cuppers has used euthyscope to dazzle the area of eccentric fixation, after first covering the foveal area. By these exercises, the acuity of the area of eccentric fixation is lowered and reduced compared to the VA of the foveal-area. And thus, eccentric fixation is converted into amblyopia with foveal fixation.

In Bangerter Pleoptophore[32]: A fully controllable device dazzles out the area of eccentric fixation while the fovea is protected by a black disc. This is followed immediately by stimulating the fovea by means of intermittent-light stimulus using small optotypes. Once the patient is able to recognise the foveal light stimulus, subsidiary instruments like localiser, centrophore and separation trainer take over.

To discuss the entire chapter on pleoptics is outside the scope of present discussion.

Visual acuity: It has been stated that the acuity of an amblyopic eye could be predicted from the position of eccentric fixation but no direct relationship has yet been established.

Steady eccentric-fixation is an unfavourable prognostic sign whereas an unsteady or wandering fixation is a favourable sign.

Pathogenesis of Amblyopia

Since the low vision of the amblyopic eye is not explained by demonstrable acquired details, it is of importance to investigate the visual function of such eyes. For, this we have:

1. Objective method — electrophysiological methods and
2. Subjective method — psycophysical methods.

In objective methods: Responses from the retina and central nervous system are registered following light stimulation. These methods are

1. Electroretinography, ERG and
2. Central cerebral response (EEG + VER).

ERG: Defective retinal functions are expressed in abnormal ERG responses. This stimulated many investigators to record ERG from amblyopic eyes. No significant difference in the ERG of normal and amblyopic eyes were recorded with single light stimuli.

EEG and VER: Herein again, though anomalies in EEG recording of amblyopic patients were reported by some investigators, others reported negative or no significant findings.

As for VER, the overall impression given is that VER responses are reduced in amplitude and are delayed in appearance in cases of amblyopia. This reduction of VER amplitude, however, cannot be consistently corelated with the degree of amblyopia.

Psycophysical Methods

Various researches have been carried out to study physical changes in retina and the retino striate - cortex in amblyopic eyes and some of the findings are as follows.

Differential light threshold: The differential threshold of retinal sensitivity as contrasted with absolute threshold has been investigated and a number of workers have found a slight elevation of the differential threshold of amblyopic eyes provided the test fields were small enough in the order of magnitude of a few minutes only.

The critical flicker frequency (CFF): In some amblyopic eyes the CFF was found elevated in the macular area relative to a peripheral area. Others found the CFF to be normal in amblyopic eyes.

The findings that the visual function of amblyopic eyes occasionally recovers partially or even completely in adults after functional loss of the good eye or in strabismus monkey after ennucleation of the sound eye, indicate that even in long-standing and deep amblyopia cases the retinostriate connections of an amblyopic eye are not irrevocably destroyed but become dormant.

Summing up: Amblyopia appears to be a cortical inhibition of the highest function of pattern vision without impairment of lower function of the light — sense and spatial projection. Though amblyopia due to an acquired lesion may occur, its incidence is relatively rare and in these cases, the visual loss is passive and irrecoverable.

The usual amblyopia in a squinting eye is active, functional and of cerebral origin. The earlier it develops the more profound it tends to be and the earlier the treatment is instituted, the greater the amount of vision that can be reclaimed.

Treatment: In 1743 Buffon[14, 36] recommended patching of the fixating eye (in a case of concomitant squint) to improve the vision in the deviating eye for according to him poor vision of the amblyopic eye was the cause of the deviation.

Once again with the concept of amblyopia as a sensory adaptation to squint, patching was resumed and has since remained the mainstay of amblyopia treatment, both for the strabismic amblyopia as also for cases of straight-eye amblyopic (anisometropic amblyopia).

But before occlusion of the sound eye, refractive error (if any) should be assessed under cycloplegic mydriasis and full refractive correction consistent with the visual comfort of the child should be prescribed. In an unilateral high hypermetropia, under-correction may be necessary.

Occlusion Treatment

Occluding the sound eye forces the child to use the amblyopic eye. In addition, it removes the inhibiting stimuli to the amblyopic eye that arise from stimulation of the fixing eye.

It appears to be a simple procedure and in many cases it is so. But the practical application of this simple procedure is beset with many difficulties, more so in young children.

There are many different ways for occluding the eye:

a. By attaching an occluder to the glass or pasting the lens with a dark black paper so that no light can get through the paper and glass to the eye,

b. By a piece of material that fastens directly to the skin around the orbit.

The important thing, however, is that the fixating eye should be occluded completely and constantly during all working hours. The child should be re-examined at frequent intervals and vision of both the eyes be noticed. Sometimes, it so happens that the vision is the fixating eye under occlusion goes down or it becomes amblyopic. This, however, is reversible and in such cases occlusion has to be made alternating, alternate occlusion of sound eye with occlusion of the amblyopic eye.

Occlusion

It has to be constant until the vision of the amblyopic eye and its fellow eye becomes equalised or until there is no improvement even after three months of constant occlusion.

· J. T. Flynn[22] *et al* (June 2000) in their extensive study of the therapy of amblyopia conclude "factors that appeared closely related to a successful outcome of patching therapy were patients age and depth of visual loss before treatment" This further supports the value of early detection and screening for amblyopia.

Marie Cleary[34] (2000) states that in terms of occlusion duration, maximum improvement occurs in response to 400 hours of occlusion wear and to full time occlusion. She further states that occlusion is more effective in the treatment of strabismic amblyopia than spectacles alone and the effect is optimal within the first six months of wear.

The visual improvement in the amblyopic eye is better in straight-eye amblyopia cases than in cases where amblyopia is associated with squint. This, however, is not acceptable in different studies.

In suitable cases of anisometropic-amblyopia, where the refractive difference does not exceed plus + 4 diopter, a visual acuity of 6/9 may be achieved. The VA may improve in these children upto the age of 15 to 16 years (sometimes even in college going students upto 20 years of age) whereas in squint amblyopic cases the visual acuity has practically no chance to improve once the age of 6 to 7 years has passed without any active treatment.

Amblyopia tends to recur until the child has reached 8 to 10 years of age because of the persistence of inhibitory effect from the fixating eye and it may be necessary to resume occlusion. Such children who are at risk of having recurrence of amblyopia, can be helped by alternating penalisation.

Sneak or slowly increasing occlusion may be tried in children between 2 to 4 years of age. In this method graded papers are pasted on the lens reducing the vision in the good eye to a known extent varying from 6/9 to 6/60. The purpose is to put the good eye gradually at a disadvantage in order to encourage the weak eye.

Occlusion in Squinting Eye with Eccentric Fixation

Many investigators are of the opinion that after two years of age, occlusion of the sound eye is contraindicated in amblyopes with eccentric-fixation, since it may reinforce the anomalous fixation behaviour. They suggest that instead the amblyopic eye should be occluded to break-up the abnormal fixation behaviour. This is inverse occlusion.

However, other workers have reported that the occlusion of the sound eye (direct occlusion) is effective until 5 years of age regardless of the fixation behaviour. To stear clear of the controversy, many now use inverse-occlusion only during the initial phase of therapy of eccentric fixation in children older than 5 years of age and then switch on to occlusion of the sound eye.

Red filter treatment: (Brinkler and Katz 1963 *AJO* 55; 1033), Malik et al *BJO/* 52-839' 1968, Rohatgi and Mohanty[46], *Proc. AIOS*, 29:117-122, 1972 for treating amblyopia with eccentric fixation.

Brinkler and Katz (1963) advocated total occlusion of the good eye and application of a Red filter (Kodak gelatin Wratten filter-wave length 600-640 mu) on the glass before the amblyopic eye. They postulated that red light entering the amblyopic eye (the filter cutting off the other colours of the white light) is ineffective in stimulating the retinal area of eccentric fixation which is predominantly a rod populated area. Thus, a suitable red filter motivates the child to use the fovea and inhibits use of eccentric fixation area.

Regular examination has to be done to keep on studying the change in fixation. Once, it has become parafoveal or central, red filter is removed and occlusion of the sound eye is continued till the VA of the amblyopic eye improves. For this treatment, the child must be highly cooperative.

Prism: To break the eccentric fixation, use of prisms base-in and base-out before the amblyopic eye in combination with occlusion of the sound eye has been suggested by various authors with varying success. Thus Duller and Brab (1969) recommended putting the prism-base out before the fixating eye in convergent squint cases to align the deviated eye with amblyopic and eccentric fixation and thereby, create conditions more favourable for foveal fixation.

A few authors have suggested using the method along with penalisation.

Back to amblyopia with normal fixation.

Pleoptics: In 1940 Bangerter[32] began systemic active treatment of amblyopia with eccentric fixation using a method for which he coined a term called the "pleoptics". Using pleoptophore (a modified Gullstrand ophthalmoscope) and under direct observation of the fundus, the eccentric-fixating retinal area is dazzled with a bright light while the fovea is protected with a disc projected onto the fundus. This is followed by intermittent stimulation of macula with flashes of light. This treatment continues until the central scotoma diminishes and the fixation becomes central.

Bengerter invented and used a few other instruments (1946 and 1955), to increase the efficacy of the treatment.

Cuppers (1956 and 1963) at Geissen used the physiological principle of the supremacy of the foveal area over the retinal periphery. His instrument is euthyscope (a modified ophthalmoscope) in which a black disc protects the fovea while the retinal periphery including the area of eccentric fixation is dazzled with bright light. A negative after-image is evoked and enhanced by flickering room illumination. The clear spot in the centre of the after-image corelates to the position of the fovea which has regained its functional supremacy over the eccentric fixating retinal area at least till the exercise continues. Use of Hadinger brushes (coordinator) completes the exercise.

But after a few years of great enthusiasm (1945-1970) the pleoptic treatment of amblyopia with eccentric fixation has waned for a number of valid reasons. Pleoptic exercises are not practical for the following reasons.

a. They can only be used in children above the age of 6 or 7 years as young children cannot cooperate sufficiently.
b. These instruments and appreciation of after image and concentration involved in the use of coordinator and pleoptophore demand intelligence which is not available in many of these young children.
c. Time-consuming and financial taxing as these exercise are, they do not appeal to parents for positive results are not many and hence, parental cooperation is also poor.

In view of the difficulties encountered in children with occlusion, an alternate method suggested is 'penalisation'.

In this method ung. atropine is used in the fixating sound eye (in order to blur vision in this eye and thereby compel the amblyopic eye to fixate at near) has been advocated often since first mentioned by worth in 1903. Combined atropinisation of the sound eye with use of miotic instilled at bed-time in the amblyopic eye of hypermetropic children was suggested by Knapp and Capobinaco (1956).

The principle of pensalisation is to decrease near vision of the sound fixating eye by atropinisation (this also decreases distance vision). The amblyopic eye with the use of a miotic drop starts seeing clearly at near distance and thus gets exercised which can improve its vision.

CAM Treatment for Amblyopia

Campbell et al[11] (1978) proposed a new treatment for amblyopia known as CAM (Cambridge stimulator). In this procedure a minimal time for only 7 minutes a day occlusion of the sound good eye and simultaneous stimulation (exercise) of the amblyopic eye with slowly rotating high contrast grating of different spatial frequencies is practised (Figs. 6.10 and 6.11). The number of sessions varies from ten to twenty at a stretch. This may have to be repeated at short intervals to sustain the improvement of VA in the amblyopic eye.

The Rationale of the Treatment

Visual cortical cells respond best to gratings of certain size (spatial frequency), orientation and contrast. As such a stimulus designed to exercise fully the majority of visual cells, should contain high contrast gratings of different frequencies and orientations. With this in mind, this instrument was constructed in which sharp-edged high contrast gratings were placed and rotated so as to occupy all orientational positions. Rohatgi and Chandra (1984)[43] presented a study report of 20 cases of amblyopia of age group 5 to 15 years using a CAM stimulator which showed an improvement of VA from FC 1 to 2 meter to 6/24 - 6/8 initially. And this could be sustained in at least half of the cases when examined two years after the start of the treatment with this instrument. The visual improvement was found to be better in emmetropes and hypermetropes (anisometropic-amblyopes) than in those of strabismic amblyopia.

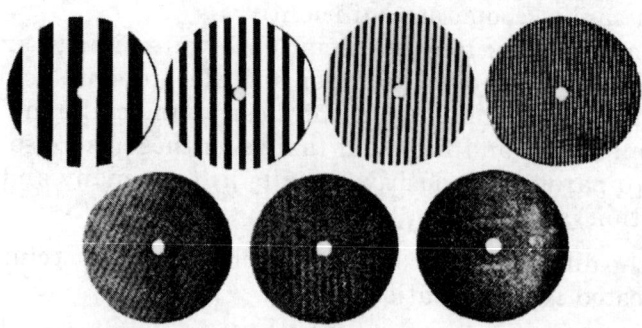

Fig. 6.10: CAM range of gratings stimuli used.

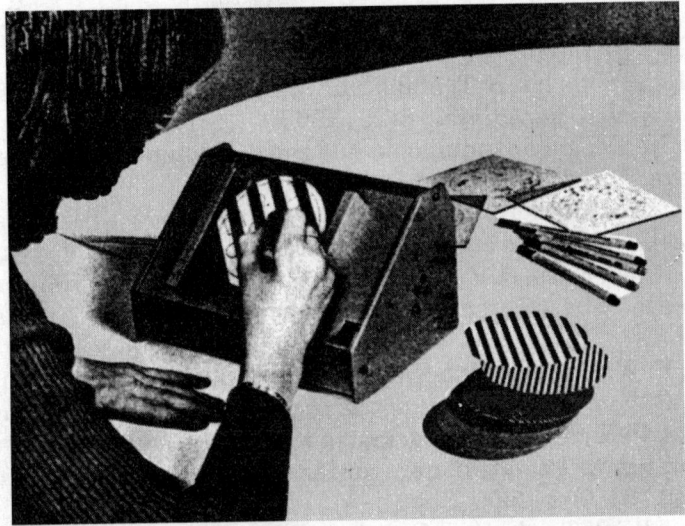

Dimensions: 270 × 250 × 250 mm   10⅝" × 9⅞" × 9⅞"
Weight: 2.3 kg   5 lb
CAM Vision-stimulator complete   Cat. No. 3.61.31480

Fig. 6.11: *A child exercising on CAM vision stimulator.*

But the finality of amblyopia treatment including those with CAM stimulator is yet not fully accepted by many authors (Mahadevan *et al*, 1981).

One would like to end the chapter by stating that though no final and unanimous line of treatment has yet been evolved for treating amblyopia-strabismic, anisometropic, vision- deprivation (amblyopia ex-anopsia) and meridional, we have the obligation to treat these cases by the best appropriate method to which one is used to, so that there is a maximum improvement of the VA in the amblyopic eye and to sustain and maintain this improvement by supportive therapy.

REFERENCES

1. Abraham, S. V: Accommodation in the amblyopic eye. *Am. J. Ophthalmol.*, 52: 197, 1961.
2. Arden, G. B., Veagan and Hogg, C. R: Pattern ERG are abnormal in many amblyopes. *Trans. Ophthal. Soc. J. K.,* 100:453, 1980.
3. Barnard, W. M. and Kelsey, J. M: Changes in the visually evoked responses during treatment for amblyopia in an uniocular patient. *Trans. Ophthal. Soc. U.K.,* 100:472, 1980.
4. Bielschowsky, A.: Application of the after-image test in the investigation of squint. *Am. J. Ophthalmol.*, 20: 408, 1937.
5. Bielschowsky, A.: Lectures on motor anomalies, visual development and causes of strabismus. *Am. J. Ophthalmol.*, 22 : 38, 1939.

6. Boeder, P.: Anomalous retinal correspondence refuted. *Am. J. Ophthalmol.*, 58: 306, 1964.

7. Brenner, R. L.: Charles, S. T. and Flynn, J. T: Pupillary responses in rivalry and amblyopia. *Arch. Ophthalmol.*, 82: 1, 1969.

8. Burian, H. M: Occlusion amblyopia and the development of eccentric fixation in occluded eye. *Am. J. Ophthalmol.*, 62:853, 1966.

9. Burian, H. M: Anomalous retinal correspondence — its essence and its significance in diagnosis and treatment. *Am. J. Ophthalmol.*, 34: 237, 1951.

10. Campbell, F. W., Hess, R. F., Watson, P. G. and Bank, R.: Preliminary results of a physiologically based treatment of amblyopia. *Brit. J. Ophthalmol.*, 62: 748, 1978.

11. Campbell, F. W. *Transac Oph. Soc. U. K.*, 99 : 326, 1979.

12. Chavasse, B. F. *Worth's Squint or the Binocular Reflexes and the Treatment of Strabismus*, Philadephia, P. Blackiston's Son & Co. Inc., 1939.

13. David Newsham: Parental non-cordance with occlusion therapy. *Brit. J. Ophthalmol.*, 84: 962, 2000 (Sept.).

14. Duke Elder, W. S: *Textbook of Ophthalmology*, Vol. 4, London, Henry Kimpton, 1949.

15. Duke Elder, W. S: *System of Ophthalmology*, Vol. 6, Ocular Motility and *Strabismus*, London, Henry Kimpton, 1965.

16. Dyer, D. and Bierman, E. O: Cortical potential changes in suppression — amblyopia. *Am. J. Ophthalmol.*, 35: 66, 1952.

17. Eggers H. M: Current state of therapy for amblyopia Trans. *Ophthal. Soc. U. K.* 457, 99, 1979.

18. Firth Alison. Y: Adie Syndorme: Evidence for refractive-error and accommodative asymmetry as the cause for amblyopia. *Am. J. Ophthalmol.*, 128: 118-119, 1999.

19. Fitton, M. H: Pleoptics in the USA. *Br. Orthop. J.* 19: 35, 1962.

20. Flynn. J. T.: Spatial summation in amblyopia. *Arch. Ophthalmol.*, 78: 470: 697, 1967.

21. Flynn, J. T.: Dark adaptation in amblyopia. *Arch.Ophthalmol.*, 79: 697, 1968.

22. Flynn, J. T.: Woodruff, G, Thompson J. R. Hiscox F. *et al*: The theory of amblyopia: An analysis comparing the results of amblyopia - therapy utilising two pooled data sets. *Trans. Am. Ophthalmol. Soc.*, 97: 373, - 290; 1999 Quoted *in Am. J. Ophthalmol.*, 12 d, 6, 831 - 832, 2000.

23. Franceschetti, A. T. and Burian H. M: Visually evoked responses in alternating strabismus. *Am. J. Ophthalmol.*, 71: 1292, 1971.

24. Helveston E. M.: Relationship between degree of anisometropia and depth of amblyopia. *Am. J. Ophthalmol.*, 62: 757, 1966.

25. Helveston E. M. and Noorden G. K. Von: Microtropia, a newly defined entity. *Arch. Ophthalmol.*, 78: 272, 1967.

26. Hess, R. F.: On the relationship between strabismic amblyopia and eccentric fixation. *Brit. J. Ophthalmol.*,61: 767, 1977.

27. Ikeda,H. and Wright M. J.: Is amblyopia due to inappropriate stimulation of sustained visual pathways during development. *Br J. Ophthalmol.*, 58: 165, 1974.

28. Jampolsky, A.: Characteristics of suppression in strabismus. *Arch. Ophthalmol.*, 54: 683, 1955.

29. Jampolsky, A: Some anomalies of binocular vision. *Proc. 1st Int. Congress of Orthoptics.* St. Louis, The C. V. Mosby, 1968.

30. Lawwill, T: The fixation pattern of the light adapted and dark-adapted amblyopic eye, *Am. J. Ophthalmol.*, 61: 1416, 1966.

31. Lawwill, T: Local adaptation in functional-amblyopa. *Am. J. Ophthalmol.*, 65: 803, 1968.

32. Lyle and Jackson: *Practical Orthoptics in the Treatment of Squint.* 5th edn. London, H. K. Lewis & Co., 1967.

33. Mai Kel Mallah, Usha Chakravorty, Patricia M. Hart: Amblyopia: Is visual loss permanent? *Br. J. Ophthalmol.*, 84: 952-956, 2000 (Sept).

34. Marie Cleary: Efficacy of occlusion for strabismic amblyopia: Can an optimal duration be identified? *Br. J. Ophthalmol.*, 84: 957 - 963, 2000 (June).

35. Nawratzki, I., Auerbach E. and Rowe, H.: Amblyopia ex-anopsia: The electrical response in retina and occipital cortex following photic stimulation of normal and amblyopic eye. *Am. J. Ophthalmol.*, 61 : 430, 1968.

36. Noorden G. K. Von: *Binocular Vision and Ocular Motility*, St. Louis, The CV Mosby Co., 1990.

37. Noorden G. K. Von: Reaction time in normal and amblyopic eye. *Arch Ophthalmol.*, 66: 695, 1961).

38. Noorden, G. K. Von: Classification of amblyopia. *Am.J. Ophthalmol.*, 62: 238, 1967.

39. Noorden, G. K. Von: Idiopathic amblyopia. *Am. J. Ophthalmol.*, 100: 214, 1985.

40. Noorden, G. K. Von and Burian H. M.: Visual acuity in normal and amblyopic patient under reduced illumination I — behaviour of visual acuity with and without neutral density filter. *Arch Ophthalmol*, 61: 533, 1959.

41. Noorden G.K. Von and Burian H. M.: The visual acuity at various levels of illumination. *Arch Ophthalmol.*, 62: 396, 1959.

42. Noorden G. K. Von and Leffler M. B.: Visual acuity in strabismic amblyopia under monocular and binocular conditions. *Arch Ophthalmol.*, 71: 172, 1966.

43. Rohatgi, J. N. and Chandra, B.: Amblyopia its treatment with CAM stimulation. *Indian J.Ophthalmol.*, 32: 436/37, 1984.

44. Rohatgi J. N. Chandra Bimal: Amblyopia in the age group of 15 to 20 yrs. *Indian Jour. Ophthalmol.*, 28, 1980.

45. Rohatgi J. N., Chandra Bimal: Trends in the management of straight-eye amblyopia. *Proc 24th Int Congress of Ophthalmol,* Rome, 1986.

46. Rohatgi J. N., Mohanty K. C.: Trends in the management of amblyopia. *Proc All India Ophthalmol Society, 29:* 117-127, 1972.

47. Scully, J. T.: Non-central fixation in squinting children. *Br. J. Ophthalmol,* 45: 741, 1961.

48. Worth C.: *Squint: Its Causes, Pathology and Treatment*, 6th edn. London, Bailliere Tindall & Cox, 1929.

49. Wright K., Edelman P.M. Walonkar, F. and Yiu S: Reliability of fixation-preference testing in diagnosing amblyopia. *Arch Ophthalmol.*, 104: 549, 1986.

50. Wright K. W. Kalonker F. and Edelman P: 10–dioptre fixation test for amblyopia. *Arch. Ophthalmol*, 99: 1242, 1981.

51. Zipf. R: Binocular fixation pattern. *Arch.Opthalmol.*, 94:401, 1976.

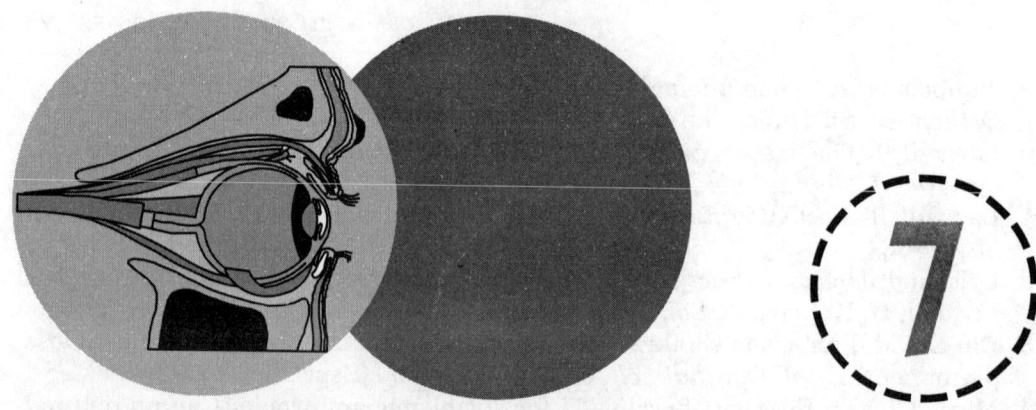

Treatment and Management of Concomitant Strabismus

7

MEDICAL

This chapter has been discussed under two separate headings (a) "Indications and principles of medical treatment", and (b) "Surgical principles of treatment and indications for surgery".

In primitive folk-lore and in mythology, squint has been and is still considered an affliction sent by an angry god and the ill-luck brought from the look of a cross-eyed person forms the basis of many legends centered round its etiology. This has, thus resulted in a wide and strongly held misconception that a child would grow out of squint with age and hence, no treatment need to be given till he/she reaches puberty.

There is a growing list of scientific studies clearly indicating that the presence of strabismus has an adverse effect on the ability of a person to perform well in school, find gainful employment and form meaningful interpersonal relationship. Strabismus creates a negative social prejudice which affects employment ability. These effects can be reversed by a successful strabismus surgery (Satterfield[34], 1993).

And thus, it is now becoming clear that these infants and young children need active and urgent treatment and at the earliest, if one aims for a full functional rather than a purely cosmetic cure.

Following are the three goals in treating and managing such cases (of concomitant strabismus).

    i. To produce cosmetically straight eyes.

    ii. Cosmetically straight eyes with equal vision.

    iii. Restoration and strengthening of the binocular single vision.

Rarely does such an ideal result occur. Usually the patient, who has had an ocular deviation, would always show some motor or sensory findings that are different from the patient who has never had strabismus.

Treatment and management of these cases is both surgical and non surgical (or medical). In vertical deviations associated with concomitant cases, it is mostly surgical, whereas in horizontal deviations it is both medical and surgical.

There are cases of concomitant squint wherein the underlying pathology is a congenital paralysis of a vertically acting muscle and which subsequently as a result of contractures and overreactions take on the appearance of a concomitant squint. In such cases, one may have to resort to surgery straightway (after necessary investigations) so that at least in the primary straight-ahead position, the patient is free from diplopia or double vision. This may be necessary in those where the compensatory head posture (CHP) has not developed on its own.

In medical treatment, the first and foremost objective is to improve the visual acuity of the deviating eye and make it normal or at least equal to the vision in the non squinting sound eye. And for this, correction of the refractive error by prescription of glasses and prisms (as and when necessary) is the sheet anchor.

Corrective lenses help in two ways

1. They create a sharp retinal image which in young children acts as a stimulus for the use of the eyes and for fusion, and
2. They help in producing a proper balance between accommodation and convergence.

Refractive Correction and Glass

Of the two types of concomitant squint cases (convergent and divergent), convergent concomitant cases are far more common. About 25% of these concomitant squint cases in children are accommodational, that is, related to uncorrected refractive error and sometimes associated with anisometropia. It is necessary, therefore, to prescribe correct glasses after a careful and accurate retinoscopy. The trend is to prescribe the full amount of hypermetropic correction including astigmatism assessed after a thorough cycloplegic examination.

On the other hand, when partially accommodative esotropia (esotropia with an accommodative element) is present, lenses are used to control the accommodative element and surgery is indicated for the residual deviation To facilitate acceptance of the correcting glass, specially in high hypermetropia cases (with or without astigmatism), it is suggested that glasses prescribed be worn while the accommodation is still relaxed (under the influence of atropine).

The refractive correction so prescribed must provide optimum visual acuity. Insisting on a correction that blurs distance vision is definitely not acceptable to the child.

As against general misconception, even children as young as 18 months of age have been found to wear glasses provided they get proper frames aided by tapes around the head.

Alan et al[2] commenting on the "outcome in refractive accommodative esotropia" conclude as follows. "Most children with refractive accommodative esotropia have an excellent outcome in terms of visual acuity and binocular single vision. Current management strategies for this condition result in a marked reduction in the prevalence of amblyopia compared with the prevalence at presentation. The degree of hyperopia, however, remains unchanged with poor prospects for discontinuing glass wear". An error of refraction may not be the entire cause of a concomitant convergent squint but it is an important predisposing factor.

After having examined each eye both for distance and near vision and prescribing the lens required to give the best visual acuity, it is important to assess for the binocular visual acuity. It may be found that a better binocular visual acuity is obtained, specially in hypermetropic cases by further addition of convex lenses in front of each eye. In such cases, it may be necessary to prescribe an overcorrection of convex lens to encourage a full relaxation of the ciliary muscle.

As for a myope with convergent squint, he may need an undercorrection of the refractive error for it is likely that the correct glass will increase the angle of deviation by causing the patient to accommodate (which he normally does not need for seeing a near object) and thus, to converge more.

Bifocals[9, 29] are sometimes useful in the following cases.

1. When it is found that with refractive correction required for distance, the deviation for near vision (reading) is not fully corrected. This may happen in those with a high Ac/A ratio. In such cases, an additional convex correction may be prescribed in the shape of a bifocal segment or as an extra pair of reading glasses.

2. When it is found that the deviation is marked only for near work and is not manifest in distance vision, bifocals may help fusional amplitudes to develop spontaneously in many such children after which the bifocals may be reduced step by step and eventually discontinued.

DIVERGENT SQUINT CASES

Fewer cases of concomitant divergent squint are controlled by the use of glasses.

It is found that in such cases (constant or intermittent in nature) where the error of refraction is hypermetropia, the deviation is usually made worse by the use of glass. Myopes, on the other hand, may need full correction with concave lenses. Rather slight overcorrection of a myopic refractive error occasionally is helpful in controlling intermittent exodeviation.

Prisms

Prescribing prisms is generally considered for cases of heterophorias or latent squint both for excercise and for treatment. Since Fresnel-prisms[3, 19] have become available, their use has increased. They are used to reduce the deviation and develop fusional amplitudes in concomitant cases. They are also suggested for use to avoid contractures of the antagonistic muscle in cases of paralytic strabismus.

These Fresnel-prisms are simply pasted to the lower part of the back surface of the spectacle lenses. They are available in power upto 30 Δ and while in use produce minimal distortion besides being light in weight. They are readily changeable and do not cause any cosmetic problem.

According to Bagolini[5], the correction or overcorrection of a residual angle of esotropia after surgery with prisms may help restore normal retinal correspondence. The improvement of anomalous retinal correspondence (ARC) with prisms raises the question whether better functional results are obtained (by converting into normal retinal correspondence) with the use of prisms than if surgical treatment alone is used.

Occlusion

Even after correcting the refractive error, there are cases where visual acuity does not improve or improves partially. In these cases one has to take recourse to occlusion of the sound eye to improve the visual acuity of the squinting amblyopic eye[17, 26, 28, 37].

It is unusual to find a marked degree of amblyopia in cases of fully accommodative strabismus partly because of a comparative late onset of the deviation and partly because of the fact that the deviation is intermittent in character to begin with. But despite the correct glasses, some degree of amblyopia may persist.

In non-accommodative cases, where visual acuity is poor, glasses may not be of much help.

In all such cases amblyopia has to be treated and visual acuity improved. And then only surgical treatment for correcting the deviation is advisable.

However, a lot depends (so far improvement of the visual acuity is concerned) on the age of the child and his cooperation as also the age when he is brought in for the treatment.

Under the age of 5 (five) years full and constant occlusion of the sound eye is necessary and may be all that is required in accommodative cases. But for children in this age group who are not cooperative, or in those who are too young to accept and wear glasses and or in whom patching of the good eye is not feasible, use of Ung. Atropine sulph 1% in the good eye and a drop of miotic drop in the deviating eye may be useful (penalisation therapy).

The sound eye may have to be occluded for at least 3 to 6 months even when on periodic examinations there is no demonstrable improvement of visual acuity (VA) in the deviating eye. Improvement of VA by even one line on a Snellen chart a month is taken as satisfactory improvement. On each visit the VA of the sound eye (the eye undergoing occlusion) must also be examined lest it becomes amblyopic as a result of disuse.

Once the visual acuity has been equalised or becomes more or less equal in both eyes tested individually, it should not be assumed that it would remain that way without some type of reinforcement. Partial or intermittent occlusion is necessary and suggested say, at least, one day a week at the weekend or at least 2 to 3 hours every day after the school hours. It should be continued preferably for a year or two depending how deep was the amblyopia (when the treatment began) till the age of 8 to 10 years. This is necessary for the inhibitory effect of fixing eye on the deviating eye may persist that long.

Thus, occlusion serves the following purposes.

a. Improves fixation and visual acuity in a deviating amblyopic eye,
b. Prevents or inhibits development of abnormal retinal correspondence (ARC).
c. Overcomes suppression and promotes alternation usually as a prelude to surgical treatment.

Occlusion is mainly carried out in children (as already mentioned) from early infancy upto about eight years of age provided central fixation is present.

In older children and college-going students (15–20 years age group) occlusion of the sound eye may also be tried to improve visual acuity in the deviating amblyopic eye. It has and may meet with some success provided the effort is not given up easily and early.

In those who show improvement of visual acuity with occlusion upto or at least to 6/60, further improvement of VA can be gained by use of Red filter (mostly in grown up school and college going children).

Red Filter

Total occlusion of the sound eye and cementing of a red filter on the spectacle glass before the amblyopic eye has been advocated (Brinkler and Kataz[8], *Am. J. Ophth.*, 55:1033, 1963) specially in those where the amblyopic eye shows eccentric fixation. The red filter excludes wavelength shorter than 640 (Kodak gelatin

Wartten Filter No. 92). The red light passing through the filter is ineffective in stimulating the eccentric retinal area (which is predominantly rod populated area). This forces the patient to use the foveal area and inhibits use of the eccentric fixation area. Once fixation becomes parafoveal or central, the red filter is removed and occlusion continues till the VA of the amblyopic eye improves.

CAM Treatment

Campbell et al[11] in 1978 proposed a new treatment for amblyopia, called CAM treatment. Details of this treatment have been mentioned while discussing the management of amblyopia (see chapter 6). The main feature of this treatment is stimulation for 7 minutes of the amblyopic eye by slowly rotating high contrast square wave grating of different spatial frequencies (see Figs 6.10 and 6.11). The sound eye is patched only during the brief period of stimulation. Stimulation is given weekly.

Rohatgi et al (1984)[32] have used CAM stimulation in 20 cases of amblyopia and followed these cases for 2 years when it was found that 50% of the cases did retain the improved visual acuity in the amblyopic eye. Many, however, are not convinced of the efficacy of this mode of treatment.

INVERSE OCCLUSION

Or the occlusion of the amblyopic eye is advocated to prevent stimulation of the eccentrically fixing point of the eye which occurs when both eyes are kept open.

It may be combined with pleoptic treatment of the affected eye or it may be used as an isolated therapeutic measure. If and when central fixation is restored in the amblyopic eye, the occlusion is changed to the sound eye (fixing eye) and continues till the VA improves.

Pleoptic Treatment

The principle of pleoptic treatment is to create a situation in which the normal fovea is shielded and the perifoveal area that is being used for fixation is temporarily blinded. This is done by using a bright light source with a shield placed in the centre of the light source so that the fovea (but not the eccentric fixation point) is protected from the dazzling light of an Euthyscope. By so doing the patient is likely to get better vision in the (normal) foveal region as it is encouraged to view objects which were so long being focussed by the eccentric area.

During the course of the treatment, the amblyopic eye is patched in between the treatment (inverse occlusion). Once the fixation becomes central and vision has started to improve in the amblyopic eye, the usual occlusion of the sound eye begins once again.

The various modes of treatment in the group of pleoptics have now been more or less given up for

1. It is not feasible in children below the age of 5 years who need it most to improve the VA of amblyopic eye.
2. Cost-wise it is very costly and time consuming.
3. And the end result in the form of improvement of VA and restoration of binocularity is not as planned.

The third perception in the management of concomitant strabismus cases, viz. restoration and improvement of binocular single vision is feasible only when it is present weak though or in rudimentary form. And herein comes the role of orthoptic exercises (Fig. 7.1).

Orthoptic Treatment

It is essentially a process of mental training in which the higher centres of the brain (which control visual sensation and ocular muscle coordination) are trained to do their work efficiently. It consists of excercises of a re-educative nature which aim at the restoration of comfortable binocular single vision in those who have deficiency of it or have lost it (as in cases of strabismus of infancy or early childhood) or in those who find its maintenance difficult as in some cases of heterophoria.

Orthoptic treatment has to be active and persuasive so that it encourages the patient to make every effort and to give all his attention.

The orthoptic treatment for accommodative convergent cases may be divided into four stages, the purposes of which are as follows.

a. To overcome suppression, particularly at the convergent angle of deviation, by active anti-suppression exercises on a synoptophore.
b. To teach the child relaxation of accommodation with consequent relaxation of convergence.
c. To teach the patient negative relative fusional convergence, and
d. To ensure that the patient has good binocular convergence. And for these the instruments used are synoptophore, cheiroscope, stereogram and prisms bars, etc.

Anti-Suppression Exercise

The idea behind anti-suppression exercise is to bring the images formed on the suppressed retinal area back into consciousness. This can be done by stimulating the retina of the deviated eye by moving the visual target on the synoptophore (major amblyoscope) back and forth across the suppression scotoma or by rapidly alternating visual stimulation of macula.

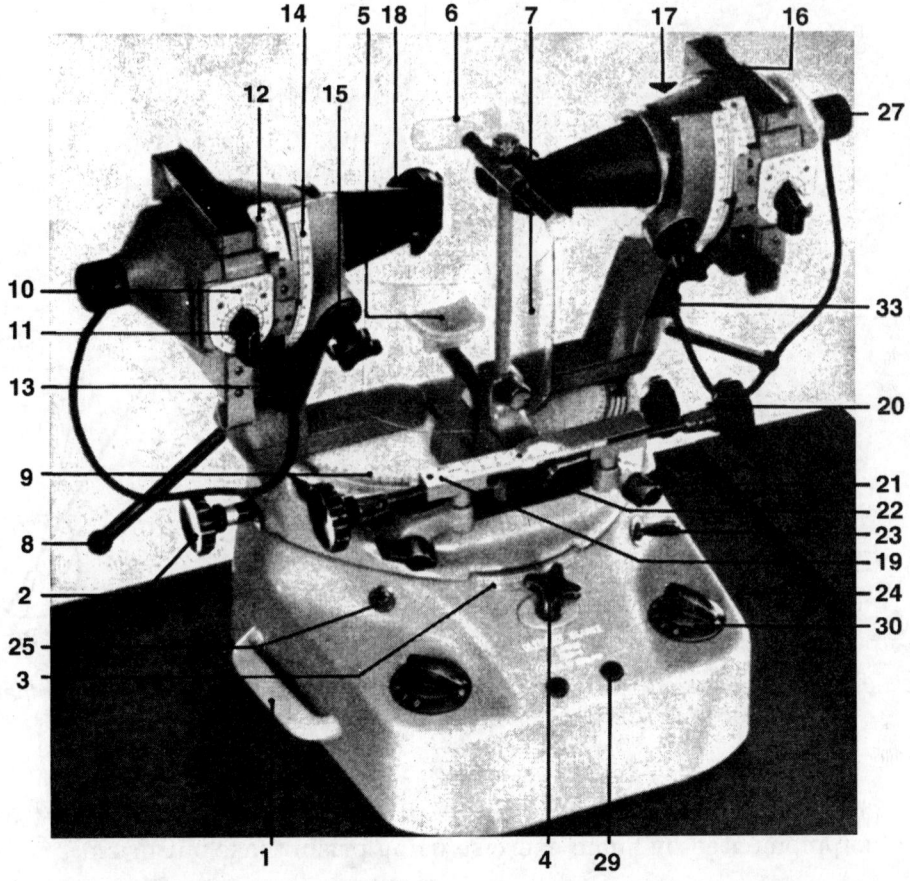

Fig. 7.1: *Synotophore for examination and orthoptic exercises.*

ORTHOPTIC INSTRUMENTS AND THEIR USE

1. Carrying handles (2), 2. Interpupillary distance controls (2), 3. Interpupillary distance scale, 4. Chinrest control, 5. Chinrest, 6. Forehead rest, 7. Breathshield, 8. Handles for adjustment of horizontal angle between tubes (2), 9. Horizontal deviation scales (2), 10. Vertical deviation scales (2), 11. Vertical deviation controls (2), 12. Torsional deviation scales (2), 13. Torsional deviation controls (2), 14. Elevation and depression scales (2), 15. Elevation and depression controls (2), 16. Slide carriers (2), 17. Slide ejectors (2) (not visible in illustration as they are on the orthoptists side of the slide carriers, 18. Auxiliary lens holders (2), 19. Horizontal vergence scale., 20. Horizontal vergence controls (2), 21. Tube locking controls (horizontal) (2), 22. Central lock, Electrical Parts, 23. On/Off switch, 24. Mains current input plug and socket, 25. Indicator lamp, 26. Voltage selector, 27. 6 V lampholders (for slide illuminator) (2), 28. 12 V lampholders (for after-images and Haidinger's brushes) (2), 29. Hand flashing switches (2), 30. Dimming rheostats (2), 31. Selector switch, 32. Plug and socket connection to Automatic Flashing Unit (Model 2052 only), 33. Plug and socket connection to 6 V lamps (2).

Before this exercise, the patient has to be made aware of his physiological diplopia as shown in Fig. 7.2. (also see Figs 3.5 and 3.6 in Chapter 3).

Improvement of fusion or increasing fusional amplitude (both convergent and divergent), This can be done on a major amblyoscope after having set the slides (targets) in the two tubes at an angle at which the patient can fuse. The tubes or the arms of the major amblyoscope are diverged or converged until

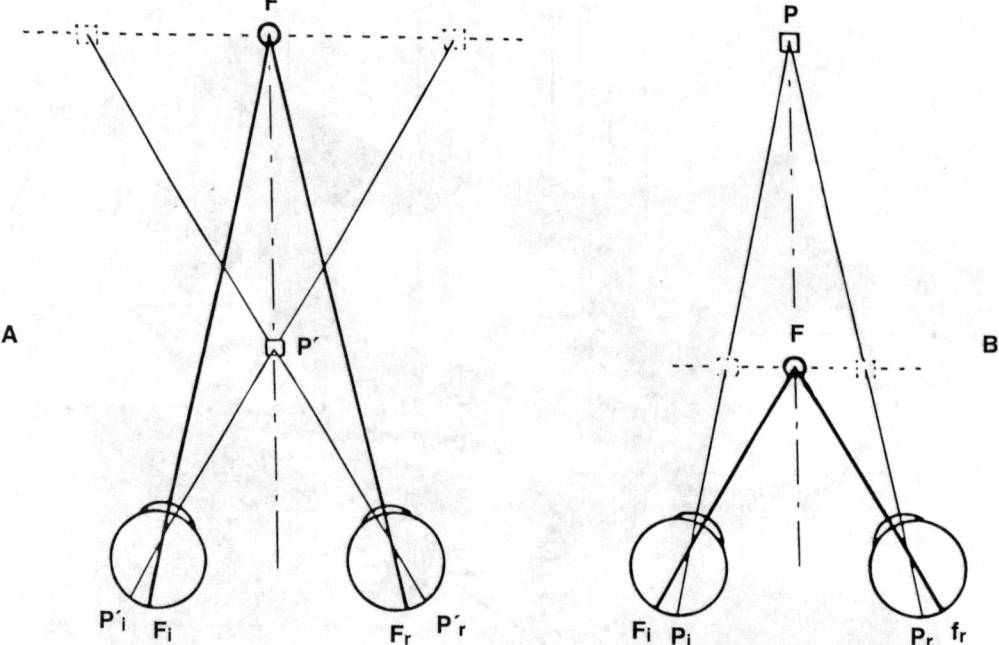

Fig. 7.2: *Physiological diplopia—crossed (A) and uncrossed (B) A-Object P closer than the fixation point F, B-Object P more distant than the fixation point F.*

diplopia occurs. This has to be done gradually and rapidly. This fusional training can be supplemented by home-exercise using prism (base out prism).

Convergence Insufficiency

This can be treated to improve the convergence. The patient is told to converge on an approaching object such as a pencil or light. And this leads to sustained convergence on near objects by decreasing the distance of the object gradually. This is suggested as home excercise.

The patient is made aware of physiological diplopia of a distant object while fixating on a near target. The near target is then removed and convergence is sustained for increasing time by voluntary efforts while diplopia is maintained at distance. This is followed, thereafter, by using base out prisms and treatment at major amblyoscope. Base out prism may also be used during reading. These serve to increase the convergence capability.

When, however, the binocular single vision is rudimentary or poor and is not feasible of improvement, surgical treatment is nearly always necessary at least for cosmetic reasons. And this cosmetic improvement is an equally important aspect of treatment of all strabismus cases.

Treatment with Drugs

The use of miotics as an adjunct to the medical treatment of strabismus was highlighted by Abraham[1] in 1949. These produce two-fold action: (a) When used as drop in eye these drugs cause constriction of the pupil. A pin-hole effect is produced, thereby enabling clear vision without any effort of accommodation; and (b) by contraction of the ciliary muscle accommodation is stimulated.

So the combined effect of the two leads to a reduction in the need for a subjective effort of accommodation to see clearly at near distance. And a reduction in the subjective effort of accommodation means less accommodative convergence, the result being that clear vision is achieved without the occurrence of a manifest convergent deviation.

These drugs are useful in children

1. Too young for use of glasses or who will not tolerate glasses or who are unlikely to wear glasses for the entire day.
2. With residual esotropia for near which persists despite the use of bifocals (as also).
3. With a residual esotropia for near objects or study, in a child after surgery when the eyes have become orthophoric otherwise. These are cases of a high AC/A ratio.

But miotics[14] have their side effects and one has to be careful about the side effect which may arise from their prolonged use.

Phospholine Iodide

A 0.03% solution of phospholine-iodide or ecothiophate is the drug of choice, starting with one drop per day in each eye. Long acting cholinesterase inhibitors such as DEF and demecarium bromide (hemorostat) are not preferred because of side-effects, both general (like nausea, vomiting, diarrhoea, abdominal cramps) and local (like transient blurring of vision and development of iris cyst).

One has to keep in mind that miotics should not be used unless some degree of binocularity can be achieved. A mere reduction of esotropia for near vision may be helpful temporarily, but the ultimate aim is to facilitate improvement of binocular single vision.

A failure to respond to miotics is a consistent feature of non accommodative esotropia and this serves as a diagnostic trial in some esotropic infants, to differentiate between non accommodative and accommodative esotropia.

Botulinum Toxin Injection (BTX)

Scott in 1970[35] introduced the use of diluted botulinum A toxin (BTX) for weakening an extraocular muscle.

Clostridium botulinum produces an exotoxin which rapidly and strongly binds to the presynaptic nerve terminals of cholinergic axons. It is thus, internalised into intra-cellular compartment where it inhibits the release of acetyl-choline. And this causes functional denervation of the muscles for several weeks. A long-term exposure to the toxin causes atrophy of muscle fibres. Of the six toxins A to F, type A is used clinically. Commercially botulinum toxin[35] is available as (1) Occulinum (Allergen Pharmaceutical), and (2) Dysport, U.K.

It is available in frozen and lypholised form and has to be or reconstituted before use. The unit is called mouseunits — not of weight but of bioactivity. The lethal dose (LD_{50}) for humans is 40 units per kg.

1 ng of Dysport contains 40 mouse units, whereas 1 ng of oculinum contains 2.5 mouseunits. The dose used in strabismus is less than 1/100 of the estimated LD_{50} for human.

The injection is performed under local or general anaesthesia and under electromyographic control through a needle that doubles as an electrode. It has been used for strabismus, blepharospasm, hemifacial spasm and nystagmus.

So far as strabismus is concerned, it has been used in the following conditions.

1. *Esotropia* Scott[35, 36] injected 261 patients with esotropia. A 68% reduction in deviation (by 10 prism dioptres) was achieved after a follow up of 6 to 65 weeks. Bigland et al[6A] found valuable results by injection of medial rectus for consecutive esotropia.

2. *Exotropia* The results are not as good as in cases of esotropia.

3. *Paralytic strabismus* One of the best indications for the use of botulinum toxin is in the treatment of 6th nerve palsy. Bolutinum is injected into the antagonist medial rectus muscle. This usually balances the paralysis and straightens the eye.

Botulinum A injection has also been used to control nystagmus besides cases of blepharospasm and hemifacial spasm, where other forms of treatment have not been successful in attenuating the deviation of the patient.

One would like to conclude this chapter by stating what Jampolsky[18] wrote in "Some uses and abuses of orthoptics — the present status" (*Trans. New Orleans Academy of Ophthalmology, 1971*). "We must continue the quest for new knowledge in strabismus diagnosis and be careful to differentiate that which is valid, useful and helpful from that which is often inaccurate, not used but interesting.

"We should know what we can do and should do. We should know what we can do, but should not necessarily do. We should know what we cannot do and therefore should not do. Wisdom comes from knowing which is which."

REFERENCES

1. Abraham S. V.: The use of miotics in the treatment of convergent strabismus and anisometropia, a preliminary report. *Am. J. Ophthalmol.*, 32: 233, 1949.
2. Alan Mulvihill, Aoife MacCann, Ian Fliteroft, Micoael O'Keefe: Outcome in refractive accommodative esotropia. *Br. J. Ophthalmol.*, 84, 746, 749, 2000 (July).
3. Aust W.: The use of prisms in pre- and post-operative treatment, In Fells, P. (Editor). Proc. *First Congress International Strabismological Association*, St. Louis, The C. V. Mosby Co, 1971.
4. Arruga A.: Effect of occlusion of amblyopic eye on amblyopia and eccentric fixation. *Trans. Ophthalmol. Soc., U. K., 82: 45, 1962.*
5. Bagolini B.: Sensory anomalies in Strabismus. *Br. J. Ophthalmol,* 58 313, 1974.
6. Bangerter A.: The purpose of pleoptics. *Ophthalmologica,* 158: 334, 1969.
6A. Bigland A. W. *et al: Experience with botulinum A Toxin (Oculinum) in the treatment of strabismus content ophthalmol form 5: 230, 1987.*
7. Breinin G. M., Chin N. B. et al: A rationale for therapy of accommodative strabismus. *Am. J. Ophthalmol.,* 661: 1030, 1966.
8. Brinker W. R. and Katz S. L: New and practical treatment of eccentric fixation. Am J. Ophthalmol. 55: 1033, 1963.
9. Burian H. M.: Use of bifocal spectacles in the treatment of accommodative esotropia. *Br.Orthopt. J.,* 133, 1956.
10. Burian H. M.: Occlusion amblyopia and the development of eccentric fixation in occluded eyes. *Am. J. Ophthalmol.,* 62 : 853, 1993.
11. Campbell F. W., Hess R. F., Watson P. G. and Bank R.: Preliminary results of a physiologically based treatment of amblyopia. *Br. J. Ophthalmol.,* 62 : 748, 1978.
12. Cupper C.: Some reflections on the possibility of influencing the pathological fixation act. *Ann Roy. Coll Surg. Eng.,* 38: 308, 1966.
13. Duke Elder S. and Wybar K.: *System of Ophthalmology,* Vol. 6, St. Louis, The C. V. Mosby Co. 1973.
14. Ellis P. P. and Esterdahl M.: Echothiophate iodide therapy in children: effect on blood - cholinesterase levels. *Arch.Ophthalmol.* 77: 598, 1967.
15. Fleming A., Pigassou R. and Garipuy J.: Adaptation of a method of prismatic over-correction for treating Strabismus in children one and two years old. *J. Pediat. Ophthalmol.,* 10: 54: 1973.
16. Goldstein, J. H.: The role of miotics in strabismus. *Survey Ophthalmol.,* 13 : 31, 1968.
17. Hardesty, H. H.: Occlusion amblyopia — report of a case. *Arch Ophthalmol.,* 62: 314, 1959.
18. Jampolsky, A.: A simplified approach to strabismus diagnosis, In Symposium on Strabismus, *Trans. New Orleans academy of Ophthalmology,* St. Louis, C. V. Mosby Co, 1971.
19. Jampolsky A., Flom M. and Thorson J. C.: Membrane fresnel prisms — a new therapeutic device, In Fells P. (Editor) *Proc First Congress of International Strabismological Association,* St. Louis, The C. V. Mosby Company, 1971, p. 183.
20. Johnson D. S. and Antuna J.: Atropine and miotics for treatment of amblyopia. *Am. J. Ophthalmol.,* 60: 889 1965.

21. Knapp P.: The Clinical management of accommodative esotropia. *Am. Orthopt. J.*, 17: 8, 1967.

22. Letson R. D.: The use of drugs in the management of Strabismus. *Survey Ophthalmol.*, 14: 428, 1970.

23. Maraini G. and Pasino L.: Development of normal binocular vision in early convergent Strabismus after Orthophoria. *Br. J. Ophthalmol.*, 49 : 154, 1965.

24. Melling J., Hambleton P. and Shone C. C.: Clostridium botulinum toxins: Nature and preparation for clinical use. *Eye*, 2: 16 - 23, 1988.

25. Elston J. Lee, Vickers, Powell C., Ketley J. and Hogga: Botulinum therapy for squint, *Eye²*: 24 - 28, 1988.

26. Noorden G. K. Von: occlusion therapy in amblyopia with eccentric fixation. *Arch. Ophthalmol.*, 73: 776, 1965.

27. Noorden G. K. Von and Atiiah F.: Alternating penalisation in the prevention of amblyopia recurrence. *Am. J. Ophthalmol.* 102, 473, 1985.

28. Noorden G. K. Von and Mllan J.: Penalisation in the treatment of amblyopia - preliminary experience. *Am. J. Ophthalmol.*, 88 : 829, 1978.

29. Noorden G. K. Von, Morris J. and Edelman P.: Efficacy of bifocals in the treatment of accommodative esotropia. *Am. J. Ophthalmol.*, 85: 829, 1978.

30. Ratin E. and Reiter E. : Results obtained with the red-filter method in the treatment of amblyopia with eccentric fixation. *J. Pediat. Ophthalmol.*, 3 : 28, 1966.

31. Rohatgi, J. N.: Treatment of concommittant squint in adults. *Proc. All India Ophthalmol. Society* ,33, 192 -196, 1977.

32. Rohatgi J. N, Chandra B: Amblyopia: its treatment with CAM stimulation. *India J. Ophthal*, 32: 436-437 1984.

33. Rubin W.: Reverse prism and calibrated occlusion in the treatment of small angle deviation. *Am. J. Ophthalmol.*, 59: 271, 1965.

34. Satterfeld D., Keltner J. L., Morrison T. L.: Psychological aspect of strabismus study, *Arch. Ophthalmol.* III: 1100-1005, 1993.

35. Scott, A. B.: Botulinun toxin injection of the eye muscles to correct strabismus. *Trans. Am. Ophthalmol., Soc.*, 79: 734, 1981.

36. Scott A. B.: Botulinum toxin injection into extraocular muscles as an alternative to strabismus surgery. *Ophthalmology*, 87: 1044, 1980.

37. Scully J. P.: Early intensive occlusion in strabismus with non-central fixation - preliminary result. *Br. Med. J.*, 2: 610, 1961.

38. Vereecken E. P. and Brabant P.: Prognosis for vision in amblyopia after loss of the good eye. *Arch. Ophthalmol.*, 102: 220: 1984.

39. Worth C.: *Squint: Its Causes, Pathology and Treatment*, 6th edn. London, Bailliére Tindale & Cox, 1929.

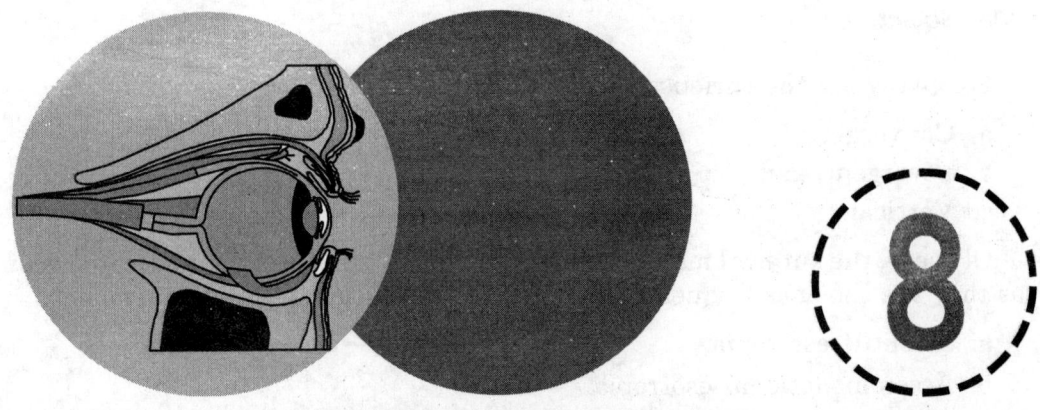

8

Surgery for Concomitant Squint
Indication and Underlying Principle

Surgery in concomitant strabismus cases aims at rendering the visual-axis of the two eyes parallel in all meridians without any conscious effort. The effect of the operation is purely mechanical, just to correct the static angle of deviation by altering the action of the two extraocular muscles—medial and lateral rectus. And once the two visual axes are rendered parallel, it is expected that the natural stimuli for binocular-single-vision would come into play This, would, not only make the eyes look cosmetically better or straight but would also help in improving the visual acuity as also the binocular single vision.

Chavasee (1939) has pointed out "Operative treatment aims at securing a great deal more than the intermittent, quasinormal and puzzling stimulation provided by a stereoscope. In his Richard Scobee Memorial Lecture, Dickey[13] (1999), while "Redifining outcomes: 50 years of decision making in strabismus management" mentions as follows: "We should not be hesitant to employ surgery when it is indicated; practically all operations devised for oculorotatory muscles are slight variations of a basic few and it is upto the individual surgeon to select the particular variation which suits him best in the light of his technique and experience."

Following are the various types of concomitant strabismus.

a. Convergent,

b. Divergent, and

c. Vertical.

Of these, the surgical management of the following needs detailed discussion as they are the ones frequently brought in for treatment and management:

a. Infantile esotropia,

b. Accommodational esotropia,

c. Non-accommodative esotropia, and

d. Intermittent exotropia.

Infantile-Esotropia

Any concomitant deviation in an infant within the first six months of life is labelled as congenital or essential infantile-esotropia. Though congenital, such cases are mostly seen in the second or third month of life. The classical clinical features are:

a. Large angle of esotropic deviation usually 40 Δ to 60 Δ prism dioptre (25° or more),

b. a normal refractive error for the age-say a moderate hypermetropia of upto 3 dioptres, and

c. normal neurological examination.

Some of these children may show alternate deviation. Associated additional findings may be nystagmus, dissociated vertical deviation (DVD), inferior-oblique overreaction and a V-exotropia.

Surgery is the treatment of choice for these cases and the earlier it is done, the better is the functional result. Surgery before the age of two years has been found to be more effective with better functional cure than when done between the ages of 2 and 4 years and/or after 4 years of age.

Some such children when seen a few years later (5 to 6 years of age or more) may show an accommodative-component. However, prescription and use of glass has not been found to significantly affect the angle of deviation. But all the same the refractive error should be corrected.

To leave such children till they grow up causes amblyopia in the deviating eye and as such a poor functional outcome, when they are operated later on.

Surgery

It could be bimedial rectus recession, medial rectus recession combined with lateral rectus resection in the deviating eye or a three muscle procedure consisting of recession and resection in one eye along with recession of the medial rectus in the other eye. Any inferior oblique over-action if evident is dealt surgically later on.

But all said and done, the results of the treatment are subnormal binocular vision, small angle eso-exotropia, microtropia and occasionally a large angle deviation which requires a second stage surgery later on.

Accommodational Convergent Squint

This is the familiar group of convergent squint cases presenting typically in the age group of 2 to 4 years. The convergent deviation of the eye varies in degrees or prism dioptres consistent with the amount of dioptres exerted for accommodation. And such purely accommodative cases account for nearly 25% of all cases of convergent strabismus.

As the etiology indicates full correction of the refractive error may and does eliminate the deviation (which is generally uniocular). For tackling amblyopia, occlusion of the good eye and thereafter, orthoptic exercises to relax excessive accommodative efforts (with consequent relaxation of convergence) and toning up of binocular single vision (BSV) are necessary for full functional cure.

Surgery is indicated in these cases only when:

a. There is a large angle of deviation not fully corrected by the glasses;
b. the deviation for distance is corrected with glass but in near vision there is a residual esotropia; and
c. when there is an associated vertical deviation like A and/or V esotropia, surgical correction of the horizontal deviation has been found to eliminate fully or partly the vertical component (of deviation).

Alternating Convergent Squint

In these cases with a large angle of deviation, more or less equal visual acuity in each eye, no significant refractive error or equal degree of ammetropia in both eyes and full alternation and suppression, treatment is mostly operative straightening of the eyes in one or two sittings.

The earlier it is done, the better is the result At least, the cosmetic blemish is gone which helps in the development of a proper psyche of the child. Further, early surgical straightening of the eyes followed by postoperative orthoptic-exercise has been shown to help a few children develop some degree of BSV (though it may be anomalous).

In the larger group of non-accommodative esotropia (excluding the secondary ones) there are no clear-cut and obvious etiological factors. Some of these may have hyperme-tropia but it is of minor degree and correction of this still leaves a fair amount of esotropia.

The growth and development of these children is normal, There is no abnormal face-tilt or compensatory head-posture to indicate an element of their being secondary to a congenital paralysis of a vertical, oblique or even horizontal rectus muscle. In some of them, the onset is traceable to birth or within the first few months of life.

On questioning, the parents may admit that the esotropia was intermittent at first and became constant a few years later. One or both parents or a close relation may have had squint but this is not always forthcoming.

In some such cases, when prescription of glasses correcting the refractive error causes the eyes to be aligned, refractive-esotropia is confirmed and treatment continues with the glasses being worn. However, amblyopia is to be carefully looked for and occlusion therapy started.

The crux of the matter, is that only a few parents appreciate the good results of occlusion for improving the visual acuity of the amblyopic eye and more often it is given up midway for one reason or the other.

A surgical correction of the deviation on the other hand, is well appreciated (by the parents). And some of them do undertake and appreciate postoperative occlusion seriously to improve the vision in the deviating eye.

Hence, herein also an early surgery is indicated. It has been the experience of those interested in squint - surgery that with appropriate surgery 80 to 90% of the esotropic eyes will be aligned with less than 5–8° (10–12 Δ) of residual squint. About 10 to 15% of these cases would need a second operation for the leftover or residual deviation in the first year of deviation and about 20 to 25% of these cases may need a second or third surgery before their teens for undercorrection and occasionally for overcorrection (exotropia), and sometimes for factors like oblique overaction with V or A pattern or DVD (dissociated vertical deviation).

Parents have to be told that their children (even if fully corrected by surgery) need careful eye examination for the next few years to monitor the visual acuity and look for any amblyopia. And this is one of the ways of asking these children for frequent and regular occlusion of the sound eye to maintain and sustain the improved visual acuity in the previously esotropic eye, Says Helveston[15]: "I tell families of infants treated surgically for congenital esotropia that they need an ophthalmologist for a friend at least until the child receives a driver's license - until the mid-teens".

The general understanding in our profession is that bifoveal fusion cannot be achieved as an adult, unless it was previously present in childhood. To this one can quote from Kushner and Morton[21] who found that 86% of adult strabismic patients developed binocular fusion postoperatively when tested with Bagolini striated lenses.

Binocularity was achieved regardless of the type or duration of deviation or the depth of amblyopia in the deviating eye. Scot et al[38] found that some type of binocularity was achieved in upto 53% of acquired esotropic adults and up to 78% of adult exotropes.

The goal of adult strabismus surgery is thus to correct or reverse a pathological condition, not simply or only to enhance cosmetic beauty. Successful surgery is associated with relief from visual confusion or diplopia, a very high percentage of sensory binocular fusion, and expanded peripheral visual field and improved psychological functions (Arthur Rosenbaum[36], 1999).

The fourth group are cases of intermittent exotropia: such exotropia may be basic, divergent-excess-type or convergence-weakness type. These cases are generally evident, between 1½ to 3 years of age.

Surgery

Surgery in exotropia is dependent on (1) the angle size of deviation, (2) the age of the patient, and (3) the state of fusional control. When the deviation is pronounced, say more than 45 Δ or 50 Δ prism-dioptre an early surgery is recommended.

Age of Patient - In young children with constant exotropia right from birth or shortly after birth and with no history of intermittency and with deviation of more than 15° (30 Δ prism dioptre) surgery should be undertaken as soon as possible after reliable measurements of the deviation are obtainable. This is feasible between 1 and 2 years of age, otherwise, amblyopia and loss of stereopsis are likely.

When the deviation is intermittent or has become constant after a long period of intermittency, surgery may be delayed and efforts directed to improve the binocular function. Efforts have to be made to eliminate amblyopia or eradicate suppression by means of alternate occlusion and by orthoptic exercises on synoptophore. In these case fusion may be reinforced with prescription of over-minus lenses (that involve accommodative convergence).

Even in these cases, when regular periodic examinations show an increase in degree of basic deviation or development of suppression during the manifest period of strabismus, surgery is indicated. And finally surgery is indicated and performed in these cases when the patient wishes it either, because of the problem of appearance or/from asthenopia or both.

The *desirable age* for surgery in cases of intermittent-exotropia is a matter of dispute. Some prefer early surgery, while others like to delay it based on their concepts of binocular function retention and reinforcement (in these cases). They have the following arguments for delaying the operation.

a. Over correction is easier to deal with in elderly children who are more cooperative.

b. Some such cases may show spontaneous correction of the deviation.

c. Amblyopia is not common in such children.

However, one thing is clear, that the excellent potential for binocular fusion cannot be sustained comfortably for long period of time and surgery is thus needed in these cases at an early age. There is a negligible chance that the condition/deviation will cure itself and a reasonable chance that it will stay the same. The majority will become worse in that the deviation will become manifest most of the time. In alternate divergent cases surgery is indicated early without losing time since alternate suppression, once it gets established, would not go easily and any chance for BSV would be jeopardised.

Surgical Details

After having considered the indications of surgery in these groups of concomitant squint, I now pass on to how surgery is done. But before surgery, a brief mention of the essential surgical anatomy of the four rectus muscles would not be out of place.

The four rectus muscles—medial rectus, lateral rectus, superior rectus and inferior rectus—originate in the posterior part of the orbit surrounding the optic foramen and in part the superior orbital fissure. The origin of these muscles is arranged in a more or less circular fashion "annulus of Zinn" (see Fig. 1.3).

All the four recti are on an average 40 mm long. They run anteriorly to get inserted into the Sclera on the surface of eyeball creating an ellipse-depicted by the "Spiral of Tillaux. The insertion is tendinous, the mean distance from the limbus being medial rectus 5.5 mm (see Fig. 1.5).

Inferior rectus	6.5 mm
Lateral rectus	6.9 mm
Superior rectus	7.7 mm

It has to be noted that the muscle insertion in the sclera is not linear. It is more or less curved and sometimes even wavy. In cases of MR and LR the line of insertion is often slightly convex towards the corneal limbus. For SR and INR, the lines of insertions are markedly convex towards the corneal limbus. Hence, the linear distance of the muscle may show variation depending from where it is measured, from the centre of the muscle insertion or from the periphery of the muscle insertion.

The length of the tendon

Medial rectus	3.5 mm (smallest),
Inferior rectus	5.5 mm
Lateral rectus	8.8 mm
Superior rectus	5.8 mm

The width of the insertion being -

Medial rectus	10.3 mm
Inferior rectus	9.8 mm
Lateral rectus	9.20 mm
Superior rectus	10.8 mm

For all these figures, the given ones are mean figures.

There is a varying range, however, which is slightly different with different authors.

Esotropic patients often exhibit a variable insertion of medial rectus which may vary from 3 to 5.5 mm from the limbus. This fact has to be kept in mind when considering recession, specially in young children. A large recession may be necessary if the insertion is closer to the limbus than 5.5 mm.

Surgery in these cases may be broadly divided into two groups:

i. Operation to weaken a strong muscle and

ii. Operation to strengthen a weak muscle.

Weakening operations are: tenotomy, guarded tenotomy, recession and myectomy (in use more for inferior oblique muscle).

A simple tenotomy of medial rectus muscle in convergent cases and tenotomy of lateral rectus in cases of divergent squint has been the earliest surgical procedure (1743 Chaveliar Jackson Taylor). The accepted operation of choice, however, is recession. This procedure prevents excessive retraction of the muscle and permits grading the weakening effect.

To help increase the efficacy of recession, the recent procedures are:

a. Adjustable sutures,

b. Faden-operation (posterior fixation sutures of Brian-Harcourt[4] of Leeds), and

c. Marginal myotomy of rectus muscles-medial or lateral.

Adjustable Sutures

This technique of adjustable sutures was at one time prevalent in Europe (1940). It has been modified and again made popular by Jampolsky[16] in USA (1978). One of its exponent in UK Peter-Fells[27] (1988) uses 2 stage operation, the first stage of operation of recession under general anaesthesia and subsequent adjustment of suture the next day under local anaesthesia. In children such suture adjustments under local anaesthesia are difficult and sedation or even general anaesthesia may be required for pulling or loosening the sutures (Fig. 8.1).

In the first stage operation, the muscle is left recessed, the number of mm dictated by conventional-surgery and the surgeon is prepared either to pull the

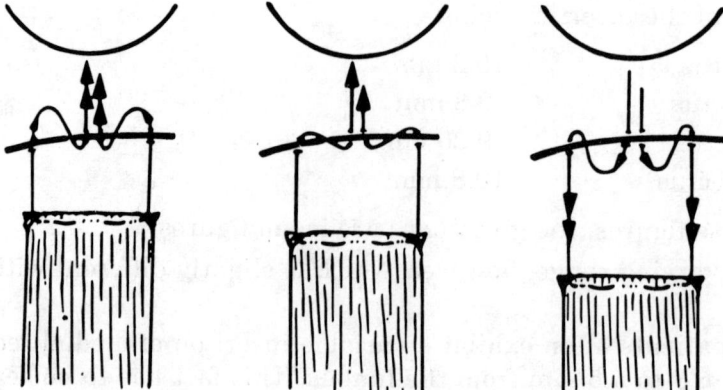

Fig. 8.1:   *Adjustable suture (Peter-Fells).*
The central figure shows the Z-shaped track taken by the suture on each side passing through the original muscle insertion.

On the left is shown one way of pulling the muscle further forwards by first enlarging the loops in front of the insertion and then by traction on the closely emergent sutures.

On the right is method for further recession of the muscle. First the loops behind the insertion are enlarged and then the patient is encouraged to look in the direction of muscle action while the surgeon holds the eye firmly by the original insertion. The muscle contracts and takes up the slack in the suture, increasing the recession.

recessed muscle forward or further recess it the next day under local anaesthesia (the second stage of operation) by pulling on or loosening the sutures.

This procedure may, however, be of help in adults, where both the stages may be done under local anaesthesia.

Abraham Spierer[1] (Tel Aviv University, Israel) in his article in *Amer. J. Ophthmol*, April 2000) comparing the postoperative result of adjustable suture surgery, when suture adjustment was performed 8 hours (group I) and 24 hour (group II) after surgery mentions as follows. "In patients undergoing horizontal extraocular muscle surgery with adjustable suture, suture adjustment 8 hours or 24 hours after surgery did not produce significantly different results". He conducted his study on 90 cases of horizontal strabismus — 40 esotropes and 50 exotropes—and the follow up period was of 6 to 40 months.

However, except for large under corrections and over corrections (which tend to persist throughout the postoperative phase) the immediate postoperative position of the globe is no different when examined 24 hours or 6 weeks after surgery and thus, adjustable sutures as practised 24 hours after surgery is not of much help in assessing the final results of surgery.

Adjustable sutures, however, may be value in some patients in whom multiple previous operations or restrictive forms of strabismus (scarring, contracture or endocrine myopathy) have added a substantial factor of unpredictability to the outcome of the operation.

Faden Operation

In 1969 Aldestein and Cuppers[11] described a new operation called Faden operation which has been more appropriately called posterior-fixation-suture (Figs 8.2 A–D) by Brian Harcourt[4] of Leeds (1988).

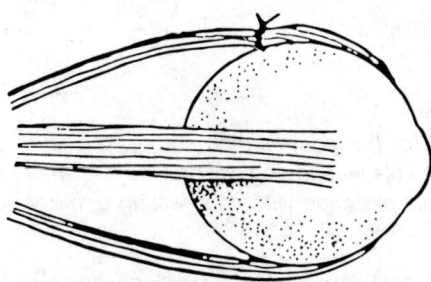

Fig. 8.2: *Faden operation. (**A**) Sutures passed through the muscle down into the sclera fixing the muscle to the sclera at a point behind the equator.*

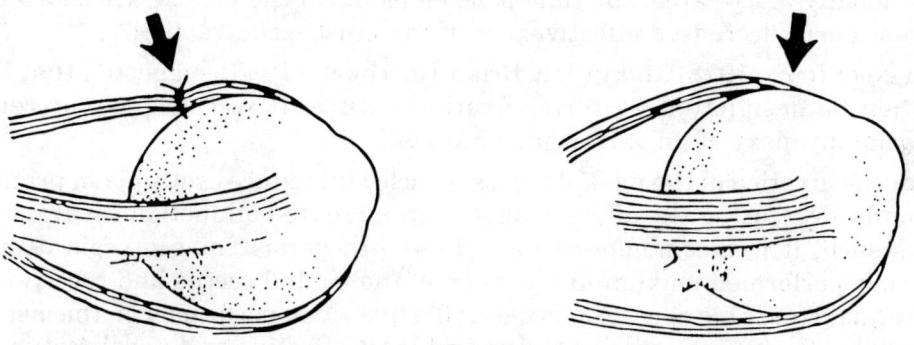

Fig. 8.2 B: *The point of effective insertion is shifted posteriorly, thereby reducing the effect of the muscle in its field of action.*

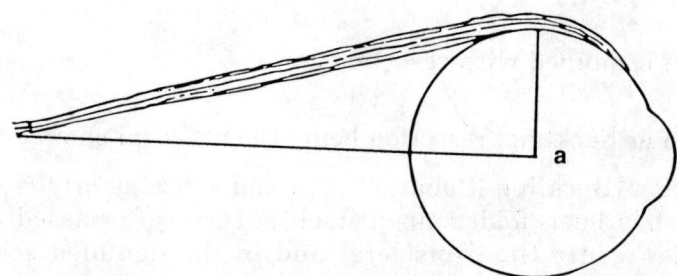

Fig. 8.2 C: *In the normal state, a rectus muscle rotates the globe by acting through a lever arm a. The muscle receives the normal amount of innervation (++) and has full range of movement.*

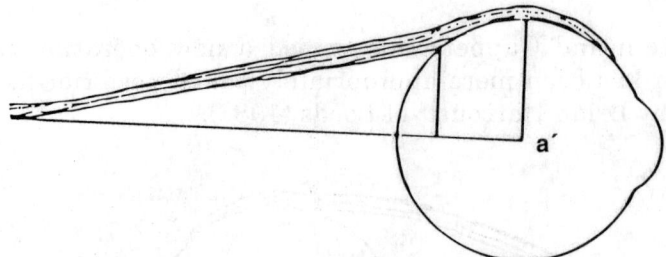

Fig. 8.2 D: *After application of the post-fixation suture, the lever arm á is reduced and the muscle is relatively weakened. This weakening will provide a form of indirect strengthening of the yoke muscle in its field of action without effecting primary position alignment.*

The operation was popularised by Cuppers in 1974. It aims to produce weakening. This effect is achieved by suturing the rectus muscle to the sclera well behind the tangential point on to the surface of the globe.

Since, the segment of the muscle between its anatomical and new insertions is functionally inactivated, the contracile elements of the muscle are shortened and this causes decreased effectiveness of the muscle contraction.

Von Noorden[23] (1978) and in UK Brian Harcourt[4] (1988) suggested that this operation be designated posterior-fixation suture. It is retropexy or retro-equatorial myopexy of an extraocular muscle.

Posterior-fixation of the medial rectus muscle will reduce esotropia in primary position by decreasing the effectiveness of an increased adduction-innervation. And as such, it is recommended in a child with persistent esotropia despite previously performed maximum recession of the medial rectus and resection of the lateral rectus. This operation is most effective when performed on the medial, moderately effective on inferior rectus and least effective on lateral rectus.

The second group of operations designed to strengthen a weak muscle includes the following:

Advancement
Resection
Advancement combined with resection
Tucking
Tenoplication or buckling, resection being the classical choice

In tenoplication (Buckling -Rohatgi[29] et al and subsequently)[32, 33, 34] after the muscle-tendon has been folded upon itself sutures are passed through the muscle-folds down into the espiscleral and in the denuded scleral tissues underneath to a depth of about 0.2 mm and biting about 1 to 1.5 mm of the sclera horizontally (Fig. 8.3 A). The author has been doing this regularly since 1958. Halveston[15] in his *Atlas of Eye Surgery* in 1973 makes only a marginal reference to this saying "I have performed too few of the procedure - plication or

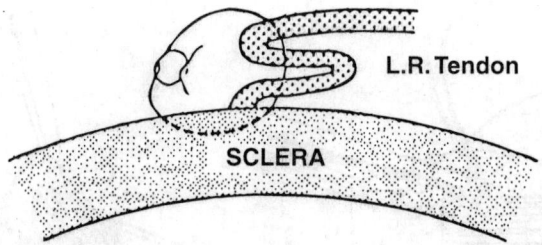

Fig. 8.3 A: *Tenoplication or buckling. After the muscle tendon has been folded upon itself, sutures are passed through the muscle folds down into the episcleral and in the denuded scleral tissues underneath.*

tuck of a rectus muscle to personally confirm this, but I believe it is true. This technique can be used on any of the rectus muscle".

Tucking and tenoplication are old methods. In tucking the muscle tendon is folded upon itself and an attempt is made to secure union between opposed flat surfaces by sutures firmly placed (Fig. 8.4). The tendon should be completely free from its sheath, otherwise the mass of tissue included in the tuck is so great that accuracy is not possible.

On the other hand in tenoplication (buckling - the author's nomenclature[29, 32, 34]) after the muscle tendon has been folded upon itself, sutures are passed through the muscle fold down into the episcleral and in the denuded scleral tissues underneath (Fig. 8.3 A). As far back as 1921 Calkins demonstrated before the American Academy of Ophthalmology the usefulness of folding the muscle and putting in sutures through the fold. He used a metallic muscle folder to produce folding of the lateral rectus or medial rectus to the desired mm. A comment by Faulkner (1944) in the *Br J Ophth* 1944 (28, 406) mentions that the muscle which was shortened by laps, folds and plication always seemed to stretch and later on showed variable results.

The operation of tenoplication or buckling has been found to be a useful alternative surgical procedure to resection in concomitant horizontal strabismus-esotropia or exotropia for the following reasons (Rohatgi et al)[30, 32].

1. The procedure has the advantage of retaining as undisturbed or at least less disturbed anterior ciliary circulation compared to the standard resection in which these vessels may get transected and which may cause bleeding while operating. Buckling operation is, thus, associated with less of bleeding.

2. This indirectly reduces the chance of anterior segment ischaemia (when three rectus muscles in the same eye have to be operated upon in one sitting).

3. Any over-correction can be easily rectified (corrected) the very next day as one has to just pull out the conjunctival stitches and thereafter adjust the muscle fold. This is obviously not possible with resection.

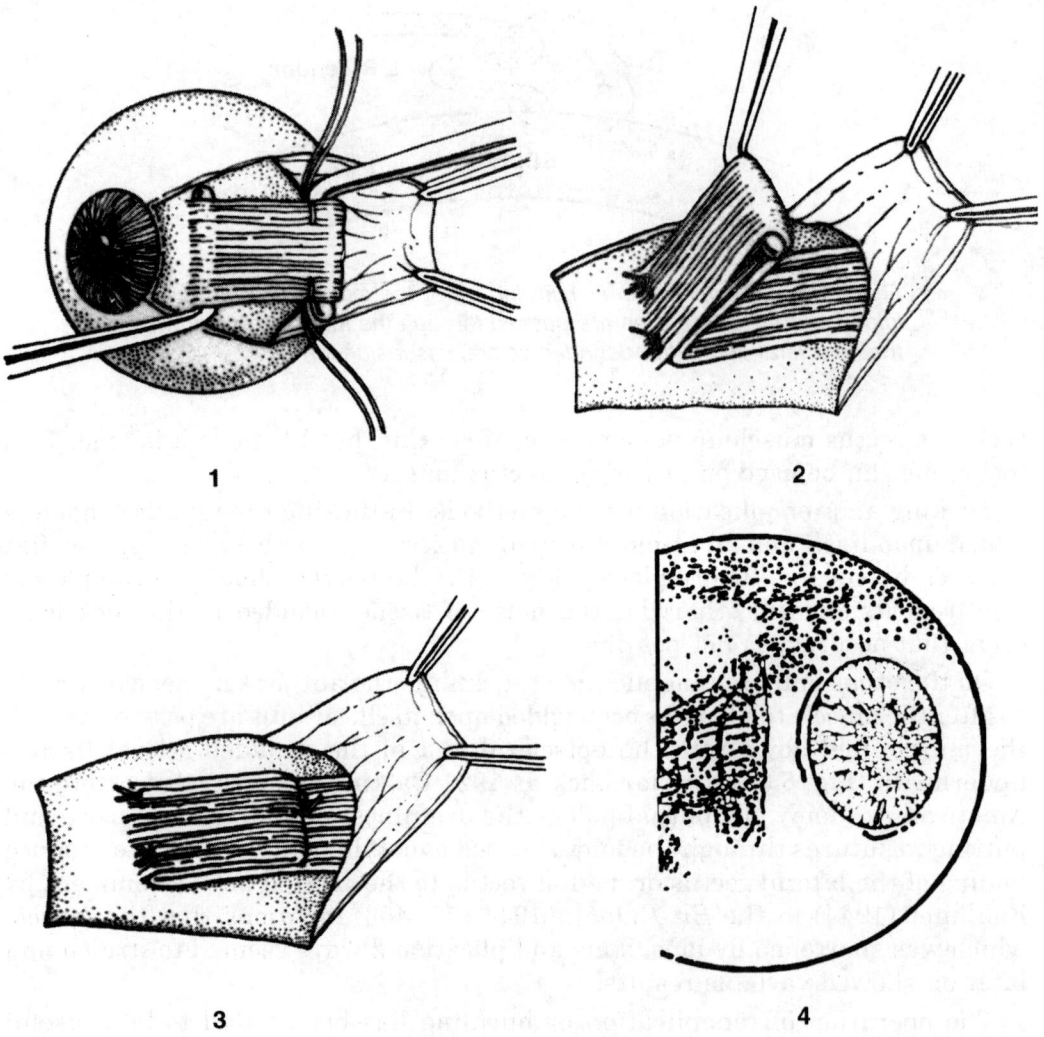

***Fig. 8.3* B:** *Photographs of tenoplication.*

1. *Steps of tucking. (i) After exposing the muscle, a double arm suture is placed at each muscle border using a locking bite. The sutures are placed a distance from the insertion equal to the intended amount of muscle shortening.*

2. *A spatula or fine muscle hook lifts the muscle about halfway between the sutures and the muscle's insertion. The needles are then passed through the tendon at the insertion. The sutures are tied, bringing the point of suture placement up to the insertion and thereby creating a loop of redundant muscle–tendon and producing shortening of the muscle.*

3. *The redundant loop of muscle-tendon is sutured to the muscle to reduce the bulk.*

4. *Raised area over lateral rectus muscle after it has been folded upon itself.*

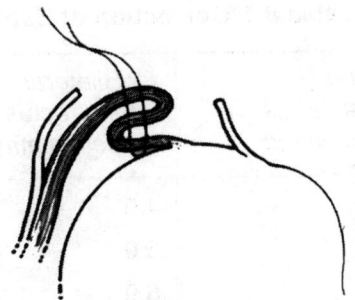

Fig. 8.4: *Muscle tucking where needle does not bite the underlying episcleral and scleral tissues.*

4. Plication, when performed carefully, produces less post-operative tissue reaction.

5. The postoperative results in our series have shown that plication is as effective as a similar-sized resection in correcting the degree/dioptre of deviation.

The amount of plication (in mm) of lateral/medial rectus is the same as the number of mm of resection, thus when 5 mm of resection is required, one would be doing 5 mm of buckling/plication of the concerned rectus muscle.

However, in some cases of plication a vertical raised lump is produced over the muscle plicated — medial or lateral rectus (Fig. 8.3 B-4). This is a sort of a nuisance and gives rise to an uncomfortable feeling to the patient and his relatives. This tends to upset the good results of the deviation having been corrected. Follow-up has shown that this lump in majority of cases gradually fades out in 2 to 3 months time.

Amount of Surgery

The exact amount of surgery recession/resection in millimetres would depend on the surgeon's experience based on a careful analysis of his previous surgical procedures. The usually followed criteria based on the experience of experts as given by Parks is as follows.

The length of recession or resection in mm is to be modified in certain situations as follows:

1. In patients with esotropia where near deviation is in excess of distance deviation by more than 10 prism dioptre, 1 mm may be added to the planned recession.

2. A patient with a large deviation will obtain greater correction per mm of surgery than a patient who has a smaller deviation.

Table 8.1 Correction of Esotropia

Deviation prism dioptre	Bilateral medial rectus recession mm	Or Bilateral lateral rectus resection mm	Or Unilateral surgery recession/resection
15	3.0	4.0	3 + 4
20	3.5	5.0	3.5 + 4
25	4.0	6.0	4 + 6
30	4.5	6.5	4.5 + 6.5
35 – 40	5.0	–	5.0 + 7 to 8
45 – 50	5.5	–	–
55 +	6.0	–	–

Table 8.2 Correction of Exotropia

Deviation prism dioptre	Bilateral lateral rectus recession mm	Or Bilateral medial rectus resection mm	Or Unilateral surgery recession/Resection
15	4.0	4.0	4 + 4
20	5.0	4.5	4 + 4.5
25	6.0	5.0	6 + 5
30	7.0	5.5	7 + 5.5
35	7.0	6.0	7 + 6
40 +	8.0	–	–

3. An esotropic with amblyopia may be overcorrected with the same amount of surgery that would produce an undercorrection in an unamblyopic patient.

4. Patients with fusion-potential should be slightly over-corrected, whereas, those without fusion-potential should be under-corrected. Patients without fusion-potential always look better with small angle exotropia compared to a small angle esotropia.

5. Before surgery, forced or passive duction test should be carefully assessed to rule out any mechanical restriction of muscle-movement. This in a cooperative patient could be carried out easily in the clinic using local-topical anaesthesia.

6. Many patients with horizontal deviation may exhibit a coexisting A-V pattern. This may be secondary to an overaction of one of the oblique muscles. A significant overaction (of the oblique muscle), however, may not exist. In these cases one would recommend supraplacement or infraplacement of the horizontal recti - MR or LR muscle and this may be enough to deflate (reduce) the A or V pattern.

The amount of supra- or infra-displacement in mm of MR/LR would depend on the difference in horizontal deviation between up-gaze and down-gaze. For, such a difference of 20 prism dioptres, the insertion may have to be moved up and down by as much as 5 mm.

A movement of the medial rectus (MR) insertion upwards weakens its effective strength, while moving the lateral rectus (LR) upwards strengthens its effectivity.

On the other hand, moving the insertion of medial rectus by a few millimetres downwards strengthens its effective strength and moving the insertion of lateral rectus downwards weakens its effective strength. The success rate of strabismus surgery is probably multifactorial. Identifying these factors may improve the surgical outcome and define the group with long term stable alignment. The surgeon should adopt the best outcome approach according to his or her own experience.

Vertical Recti Muscles

Before embarking on surgery for superior rectus muscle and inferior rectus muscle, the two vertical extra ocular muscles of the eye-ball, one has to be careful of the close relationship that exists between the superior rectus muscle and the levator palpebrae superior is and between the inferior rectus muscle and the lower eyelid. Recession of the superior rectus muscle causes retraction of the upper lid and resection may cause ptosis of the upper lid. On the other hand, recession of the inferior rectus muscle may produce drooping of the lower lid while its resection may cause elevation of the lower lid.

Surgery on the vertical rectus muscles is more effective in terms of mm of recession or resection per prism dioptre correction of the deviation than a comparable procedure on the horizontal rectus muscles.

Thus, a usual maximum 5 mm recession or resection of a vertically acting rectus muscle will produce upto 15 Δ of deviation-reduction in the primary position and slightly more in the field of action of the muscle.

In the surgical management of dissociated vertical deviation (DVD), the superior rectus may be recessed as much as 8 to 9 mm. This may be asymmetrical large recession of the superior recti. In one eye it may be 7 mm and in the other it may go up to 8 to 9 mm. And in the treatment of endocrine myopathy, a larger recession of the inferior rectus muscle of upto 6 mm or more may be alright.

Oblique Ocular Muscles

According to Helveston[15] (1993), the superior oblique is the most frequently affected muscle in acquired extraocular muscle palsy but most of the surgical activity on the oblique muscles occurs with the inferior oblique.

Myectomy or recession to weaken the inferior oblique muscle is the most commonly performed oblique muscle surgery. Overactivity or overaction of inferior oblique muscle results from:

(a) Paralysis of ipsilateral superior oblique muscle — traumatic or otherwise.

(b) Paralysis of the contralateral superior rectus muscle mostly congenital, and

(c) Primary or associated overaction of the inferior oblique in cases of esotropia. In the adducted position of the eyes, the inferior oblique muscle has its maximum action and thus, the adducted esotropic eye moves up causing up and in deviation of the eyeball elevation in adduction which may produce an A – esotropia.

There are two reasons why the inferior oblique muscle is the muscle of choice for weakening procedure in superior oblique palsy. The first and important reason is to avoid strengthening of the superior oblique because the reflected tendon of the superior oblique muscle has limited (potential) amount of slac or redundancy specially in acquired superior oblique palsy. Further a superior oblique tuck although helps in reducing the hypertropia, may aggravate the psuedo-Brown syndrome.

The second reason is that weakening of inferior oblique muscle is simple and effective.

The commonly used weakening techniques include myectomy, recession and anterior transposition as also disinsertion. Anterior transposition and myectomy were compared to evaluate the surgical result in inferior oblique by Byung-Moo et al[7] 1999. They concluded that anterior transposition appeared to be more effective in eliminating the overaction of inferior oblique muscle. But the majority of squint surgeons hold the view that myectomy is simple to perform and is more effective in reducing the overaction.

Anterior transposition of the inferior oblique muscle however, is indicated when its overaction causes excess elevation in adduction and a V-pattern in association with dissociated vertical deviation (DVD). The most likely reason for the reduction of the DVD is the mechanical or tethering effect of the newly placed inferior oblique as the surgery shifts the inferior oblique insertion adjacent and just anterior to the ipsilateral inferior rectus muscle.

A myectomy of the inferior oblique through a conjunctival incision in the infero-temporal quadrant gives the most predicatable results. It is highly effective and technically simple. And thus it is the operation of choice and preference to recession and disinsertion (Fig. 8.5 A and 8.5 B).

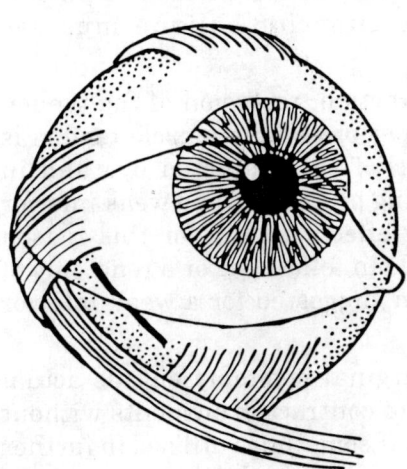

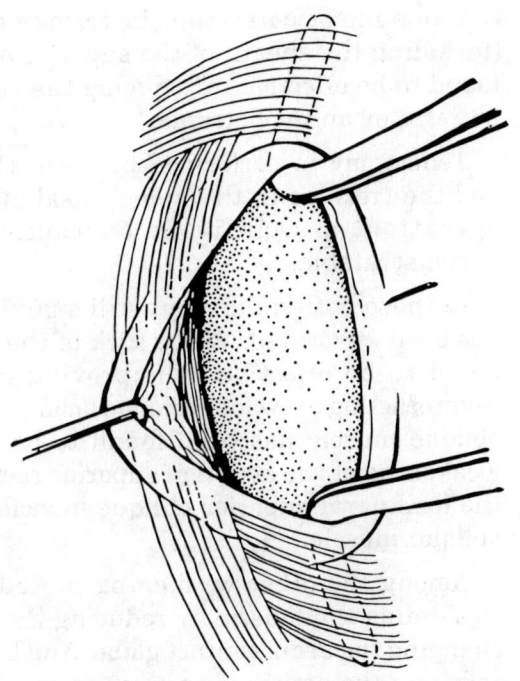

Fig. 8.5 A: *Inferior oblique myectomy. The incision for exposure of the inferior oblique muscle is approximately 8 mm long. It is located 9 mm from and is concentric with the limbus, and must be anterior to the inferior fat pad.*

Fig. 8.5 B: *To observe the anterior border of the inferior oblique muscle, the surgeon places a large muscle hook behind the insertion of the lateral and the inferior rectal muscles. A third muscle hook is used to elevate the posterior tip of the conjunctiva – Tenon's capsule incision. Deep in the incision at the junction of the sclera and posterior tenon's capsule, the anterior border to the inferior oblique will be seen.*

The average reduction of a hyperdeviation by inferior oblique myectomy in the field of action of this muscle in primary position and in the field of action of a paretic superior oblique is 11.5 Δ. This effect increases with the size of the preoperative deviation.

Recession of inferior oblique can be graded and is especially useful in cases where a minimal amount of weakening is required. Because the new inferior oblique insertion is placed at a special point on the globe, subsequent operations are easier to perform than after myectomy or disinsertion. Disinsertion has been totally given up.

Superior Oblique Muscle

An overacting superior oblique can be effectively weakened by recession, tenotomy or tenectomy of its tendon. It is difficult, however, to precisely predict the amount of correction in terms of prism dioptre achieved by tenectomy (including the sheath of the superior oblique muscle). This operation has been found to be effective in reducing the vertical deviation in downward gaze a, A-pattern, or an incylotropia.

Tenectomy is performed between the insertion of superior oblique muscle and the trochlea in the upper nasal quardrant. But before embarking on this operation, a significant overaction of the superior oblique must be demonstratable.

In those with milder but still significant overaction, recession of the tendon has been advocated. While tuck of the weak superior oblique muscle tendon is found to be effective in improving depression of the adducted eye and in counteracting excyclophoria, no such strengthening procedure for a weak inferior oblique muscle has been found to be clinically effective. And for this reason weakening of the action of superior rectus muscle in fellow eye or a tenotomy of the ipsilateral superior oblique muscle has been suggested for a weak inferior oblique muscle.

Among the other weakening procedures, marginal myotomy entails actual weakening the muscle by reducing the number of contractile elements without changing the arc of contact globe. And hence, this is sometimes utilised in further reducing the action of an already maximally recessed muscle.

Amongst the strengthening procedure for horizontal rectus muscles, one would like to mention once again the effectiveness of tenoplication or buckling. This operation as already mentioned, has been found to be easier to perform with less operative trauma and less bleeding at the operation-table (with consequent no postoperative haematoma at the site of muscle resection). But the greatest advantage is that any overcorrection of the deviation could easily be undone (the very next day) which is not feasible with the classical recession-resection operation.

Suture Material

A few words about the suture material used in squint surgery would not be out of place.

For stitching the conjunctiva, after the muscle has been tackled, 6 zero silk is still very much in use, the suture being continuous or interrupted. It is generally removed on the 4th day of operation.

Absorbable sutures: Catgut and or collagen-plain or chromic has replaced silk-suture for extraocular muscle surgery. The suture varies in size from 4 zero to 6 zero. Collagen suture has better tying qualities than catgut.

The absorption property of chromic-suture tends to make it a bit stronger and long-lasting than plain suture of the same size and hence many surgeons still prefer to use chromic material for recession or resection.

Of late, synthetic absorable suture - Vicryl 6 zero (Polyglactin 910) has become more popular for use in recession or resection of the recti muscles. It has a tensile strength close to that of silk, nylon or dacron suture of comparable size. It has longer absorption time of nearly three weeks and causes less tissue reaction. A spatulated flat needle with cutting edges and sharp point anteriorly is preferable for it produces a lamellar scleral tract of 1.5 mm or larger at a depth of 0.2 mm or deeper if need be.

Conjunctival Incision

The two commonly used procedures (Fig. 8.6 A, 8.6 B and 8.6 C) are:

(a) The classical transconjunctival incision (swan), just posterior to muscle-insertion approximately 7 to 9 mm posterior to the limbus. The vertical length is 15 mm — a couple of millimetres above and below the muscle border.

(b) The limbal conjunctival incision popularised by Von Noorden[23] (1968) which is said to provide a maximum exposure of the muscle and is associated with less complication.

A third one, self-closing transconjunctival incision in the cul de sac in which incision in the fornix conjunctiva as developed by Park (1968) is made near the appropriate cul de sac. It is suitable when the inferior oblique is being tackled, when incising the conjunctiva in the inferior temporal quadrant would do.

Some surgeons advocate a 360 degree peritomy incision when doing a Jensen (1964) or OConnor (1921) muscle transfer procedure. But this procedure may

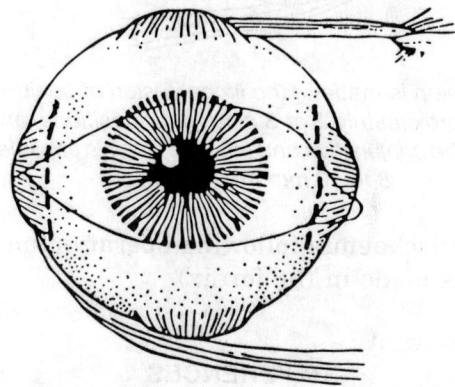

Fig. 8.6 A: *Conjunctival incision. The transconjunctival incision of Swan is made slightly behind the insertion of the medial or lateral rectus muscle (6.5 mm from the limbus for medial rectus exposure and 7.9 mm from the limbus for lateral rectus exposure) and is as wide as the muscle itself (approximately 10 mm). This incision is seldom used today.*

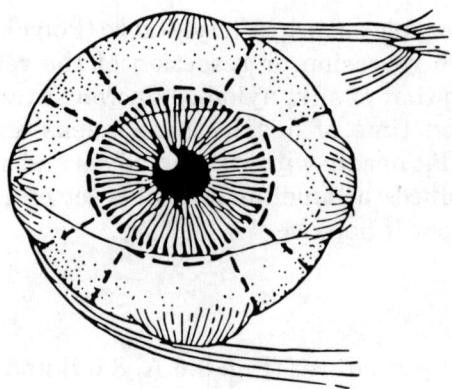

Fig. 8.6 B: *The cul-de-sac incision is made approximately 4 mm above or below the limbus and extends approximately 8 mm medially from the junction of the middle and the medial thirds of the cornea for medial surgery and 8 mm lateral from the junction of the middle and lateral third of the cornea for lateral surgery.*

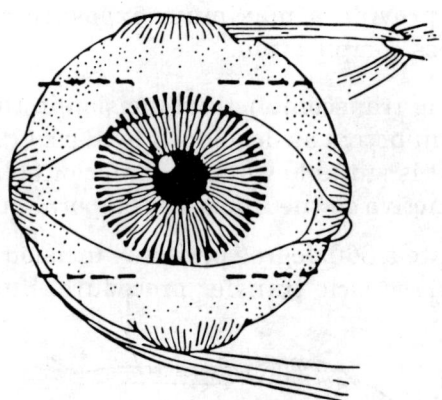

Fig. 8.6 C: *The limbal incision is made at the limbal fusion of conjunctiva and anterior Tenon's capsule and extends for approximately 2 or 3 clock hour positions, and then two radial relaxing incisions are made through the conjunctiva and anterior Tenon's capsule, extending approximately 8 to 10 mm from the limbus.*

cause anterior segment ischaemia following operation on three muscles in one sitting (when incision is made in the fornix).

REFERENCES

1. Abraham S.: Adjustment of sutures 8 hours or 24 hours after strabismus surgery. *Am. J. Ophthalmol.*, 129: 524, 2000 (April).
2. Apt L. and Isenberg S.: Eye position of strabismus patients under general anaesthesia *Am. J. Ophthalmol.*, 80: 574, 1977.

3. Berg P.: The Chevalier Taylor and his operation. *Br. J. Ophthalmol.*, 57: 667, 1967.

4. Brian Harcourt: Faden operation (post fixation sutures). *Eye* 2: 36-40, 1988.

5. Brown H. W.: Complications of the surgical management of strabismus. In Haik, G. M. (Editor). *Strabismus Symposium of the New Orleans Academy of Ophthalmology.* St. Louis, C. V. Mosby Co, 1962.

6. Buckley E. G. and Meekins B. B.: Faden-operation for the management of complicated incomitant vertical strabismus. *Am. J. Ophthalmol.*, 105: 304, 1988.

7. Byung-Moo Min: Ju-Hee Park, Seung Young Kim Seong Bok Lee: Comparison of inferior oblique weakening by anterior transposition or myectomy — a prospective study of 20 cases. *Br. J. Ophthalmol.*, 82: 206, 1999 (Feb).

8. Caldeira J. A.: Graduated recession of the superior oblique muscle. *Br. J. Ophthalmol.*, 59: 553, 1975.

9. Calkins J. W. : A muscle folder for strabismus. *Am. J. Ophthalmol.* 6, 910, 1923.

10. Cassin B., Serian4ni N. and Romano, P.: The change in ocular alignment between the 1st day and six weeks following eye muscle surgery. *Am. Orthop. J.,* 38: 99, 1986.

11. Cuppers C.: The so-called "Faden-operation" (surgical correction by well defined changes in the arc of contact), In Fells P. (Ed.) *Proc. Second Congress of International Strabismological Association*, Marseilles, Diffusion Generale de Libraire, 1976.

12. Dan De Angelis, Inas Makar and Stephen P. Kraft: Anatomic variation of inferior oblique muscle: A potential cause of failed inferior oblique weakening surgery. *Am. J. Ophthalmol*, 128: 485-488. 1999 (July).

13. Dickey F., Richard G. Scobee Memorial Lecture. Redefining outcomes: fifty years of decision-making in strabismus management. *Am. J. Orthop.*, 49: 47-60, 1999.

14. Dyer J. N.: Tenotomy of the inferior oblique muscle at its scleral insertion *Arch. Ophthalmol.*, 68: 176, 1962.

15. Helveston E. M.: *Surgical Management of Strabismus: An atlas of strabismus surgery*, 4th edn. St. Louis, C. V. Mosby Co. p. 192, 1993.

16. Jampolsky A.: Adjustable strabismus surgical procedures: In *Symposium on Strabismus:, Trans. New Orleans Academy of Ophthalmology*, St. Louis, C. V. Mosby Company, p. 231, 1978.

17. Jeong-Min Hwang, Bong Lenn Chang: Combined effect of Interceed and 5-fluouracil on delayed adjustable strabismus surgery. *Br. J. Ophthalmol.*, 83: 788 - 791, 1999 (July).

18. Keenan J. M., Willshaw H. E.: Outcome of strabismus surgery. Congenital esotropia. *Br. J. Ophthalmol.*, 76: 342-345, 1992.

19. Keenan J. M., Willshaw H. E.: The outcome of strabismus surgery in childhood esotropia. *Eye*, 341-345, 1993.

20. Keenan, J. M., Willshaw, H. E.: The outcome of strabismus surgery in childhood exotropia. *Eye*[8]: 632-37, 1994.

21. Kushner B., Morton G.: Post-operative binocularity in adults with long standing strabismus. *Ophthalmology*, 99: 316-319 (1992).

22. Noorden G. K. Von: The Limbal approach to surgery of the rectus muscle. *Arch. Ophthalmol.*, 80: 94, 1968.

23. Noorden G. K. Von: Posterior fixation suture in strabismus surgery, In *Symposium on Strabismus*; *Trans. New Orleans Academy of Ophthalmology.* St. Louis, The C. V. Mosby Co, p 307, 1978.

24. Noorden G. K. Von: *Binocular Vision and Ocular Motility*, 4th edn., St. Louis, The C. V. Mosby Co, 1990.

25. Parks M. M.: Fornix incision for horizontal rectus muscle surgery. *Am. J. Ophthalmol.*, 65: 907, 1968.

26. Parks M. M.: The overacting inferior oblique muscle. *Am. J. Ophthalmol.*, 77: 787, 1974

27. Peter Fells: Adjustable sutures. *Eye*, 2: 33 - 35, 1988.

28. Robert A. Sheriwin J., Arthur L. and Joseph L.: Posterior fixation sutures a revised mechanical explanation for the faden operation based on rectus extraocular muscle pulleys. *Am. J. Ophthalmol.*, 128: 702 - 714, 1999 (Dec.).

29. Rohatgi, J. N.: Tenoplication (buckling) as a surgical procedure in squint surgery. *Proc. All India Ophthalmol. Society*, p 320, 1966.

30. Rohatgi J. N.: Limbal insertion distance and width of the horizontal recti tendon in cases of concomitant squint. *Indian Jour. Ophthalmol.*, 29, No.4, December, 1981.

31. Rohatgi J. N.: Technique and indications for surgery of the inferior oblique muscle. *Indian Jour. Ophthalmol.* Vol 31, 1983.

32. Rohatgi J. N.: Tenoplication or buckling a surgical procedure in concomitant horizontal strabismus. *Acta Concilium Ophthalmologicum*, 1974. Vol. 2, Page 899-903, Masson Paris, 1976.

33. Rohatgi J. N.: Surgical procedure in concomitant horizontal strabismus Paper presented at 26th Int Congress of Ophthalmology, Singapore, March, 1990.

34. Rohatgi J. N.: Strengthening procedures in concomitant squint - analysis of tenoplication or buckling: Paper presented at 27th *Int. Congress of Ophthalmol.*, Toronto, Canada, 1994.

35. Romano P. and Gabriel L.: Intraoperative adjustment of eye muscle surgery. Correction based on eye position during general anaesthesia. *Arch. Ophthalmol.*, 103; 351, 1985.

36. Rosenbaum A.: The goal of adult strabismus surgery is not cosmetic. Editorial in *Arch. Ophthalmol.*, 117 Feb 1999.

37. Satterfield D., Keltner, J., Morrison T. Psychosocial aspect of strabismus study. *Arch. Ophthalmol.* 111:10-1105 (1993).

38. Scott W., Kutschke P., Lee W.: Adult strabismus. *J. Pediat Ophthalmol Strabismus*, 32; 348-352, 1995, from *Arch. Ophthalmol* 117 Feb 1999-Editorioal - Rosenbaum A.

39. Toosi, S. H. and Noorden, G. K. Von: Effect of isolated inferior oblique myectomy in management of superior oblique palsy. *Am. J. Ophthalmol.*, 88: 602, 1979

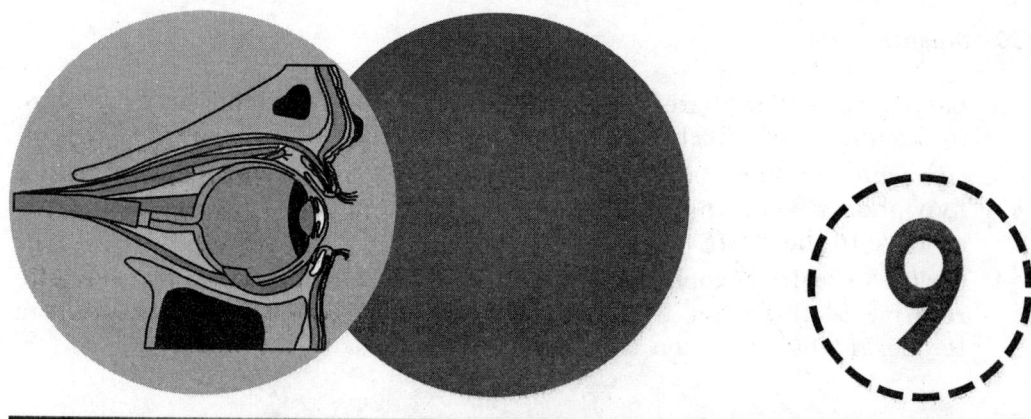

Heterophoria
Latent Squint

Heterophoria or latent squint is a clinical condition in which there is a tendency for the eyes (in their conjugate movement) to deviate from their normal relative position. This tendency, however, is normally kept in check, under stress, by the fusion mechanism (or the desire for binocular single vision). On the other hand, in heterotropia, there is a manifest deviation of the visual axis resulting from the failure of this mechanism.

Orthophoria indicates that the extraocular muscles are always in a state of perfect equilibrium. Whenever an object is viewed at any distance, both the visual axis continue to be accurately directed to that object, there being no deviation at all (except the movements for convergence and divergence).

Such an orthophoria is an ideal condition and can only be seen in deep sleep when the eyes take up a position of rest-slight divergence with slight elevation.

The relative position of the visual axis of the two eyes is determined by the equilibrium or disequilibrium of forces that keep the eyes properly aligned and of forces that disrupt this alignment. Both heterophoria and heterotropia indicate a lack of harmony between the desire for binocular single vision and the neuromuscular mechanism responsible for maintaining it. Heterophoria can be of the following types.

HETEROPHORIA

Types of Heterophoria

1. *Esophoria* In esophoria there is a tendency for one eye to turn inwards relative to the other and which is held in check by fusional impulses.

2. *Exophoria* Herein there is a tendency for one eye to turn outwards relative to the other and which is held in check by fusional impulses.

3. *Hyperphoria* There is the tendency for one eye to turn upwards and hypophoria wherein there is tendency for one eye to turn downwards relative to the other.

4. *Cyclophoria* In cyclophoria there is tendency for one eye to wheel-rotate relative to the other Nasalwards wheel rotation is incyclophoria and temporal wheel rotation is called excyclophoria.

Esophoria

Esophoria *could be*

a. Convergence excess type wherein the deviation for near fixation is as great or even greater than that for distant fixation.

b. Divergence weakness type wherein the distance deviation is smaller than that for near fixation.

Exophoria

Is commonly of the following types:

a. *Divergence-excess type*-wherein the deviation for distance fixation is greater or greater than that for near fixation.

b. *Convergence-weakness type*, when deviation for near fixation is less than for distance fixation.

Hyperphoria

A small degree of 1 Δ or 2 Δ may be seen associated with exophoria or esophoria. Larger hyperphoria is generally incomitant.

In heterotropia, or concomitant squint, the deviation of one eye relative to the other is manifest and necessary neuromuscular effort to overcome this deviation of the visual axis is not available. A case of latent deviation can breakdown for one reason or the other and the deviation becomes manifest from heterophoria to heterotropia. Cases can be seen in which there is latent squint or heterophoria for near fixation and manifest deviation or heterotropia for the distance in the same patient, or vice versa but such cases are rare.

Symptomatology

Virtually everyone has heterophoria but only a few experience the symptoms. The appearance of these symptoms depend on the state of the sensori-motor system, use made of the eyes and the general well-being of the person. The absolute amount of the heterophoric deviation is not the (most) important factor. What matters, however, is the presence or absence of a discrepancy between the amount of deviation and the amplitude of motor fusion (available neuro-muscular power).

Factors which may predispose to decompensation of heterophoria and thus cause symptoms are as follows.

i. Poor general health as in chronic or long continued illness.
ii. Continued overwork specially close work as in students burning midnight oil at the time of examination.
iii. Mental anxiety and worry or the psychological make up (of the youngman).

Symptoms These could be grouped into the following three groups.

(a) Symptoms due to muscular fatigue, resulting from the continued use of the eyes when the neuromuscular effort fails to meet this increased demand. This happens commonly following a debilitating disease. Such asthenopic symptoms may manifest as:

Eyeache with or without headache as with prolonged periods of reading, watching a film or video.

Difficulty in changing the focus (accommodating) for near object after looking in the distance or vice-versa, intolerance to bright light or photophobia.

(b) Symptoms due to failure to maintain constant binocular single vision. These may be

i. Blurring of print or running together of the words while reading which adds to asthenopia and headache.
ii. Intermittent diplopia resulting from a temporary manifest deviation of the visual axis. This occurs under conditions of fatigue and debility.

(c) Symptoms due to defective postural sensation transmitted from the ocular muscles as a result of alteration of muscle tonus. This causes difficulty in judging distances and position specially of moving objects. In case of a pilot-esophoria may cause a tendency to fly into the ground when landing and exophoria to "hold off too high".

It is the defective stereopsis which accounts for difficulty in visual judgement in some pilots when landing aircrafts. This may also occur in those doing precision tool work and in those using binocular microscopes.

Etiology

The various etiological factors that may throw the neuromuscular mechanism out of gear and cause symptoms could be.

a. *Static heterophoria*: In this condition the topographical relationship of the eyes is abnormal so that their free movements are impeded by structural factors.

b. *Kinetic heterophoria:* In this condition the synergy between accommodation and convergence is upset or disturbed and,

c. *Neurogenic heterophoria:* In this disorder the motor taxis of the eye is thrown out of gear by weakness, hyperexcitability or incoordination of the neuromuscular mechanism for it.

Static Heterophoria

The position of the eyes and the freedom of their movements to a greater extent is dependent on a number of anatomical factors. An asymmetry of the orbit, abnormalities in their inclination or in the shape of the skull (oxycephaly) or anomalies in the state of eyes (prominent eyes of high myopia) may cause a limitation of the ocular movement. Proptosis, enophthalmos or disalignment by a spacetaking lesion in the orbit or injury to orbital floor may impede or restrict the coordinated movement and thus, cause heterophoria.

Kinetic or Accommodational Heterophoria

Majority of the cases of muscular imbalance are due to a dissociation of the normal relationship between accommodation and convergence.

In the interest of clear vision, an increased demand for accommodation in moderate degrees of hypermetropia, in emmetropia associated with too much of near work or at the onset of presbyopia may lead to a tendency for development of esophoria.

On the other hand, exophoria tends to develop in congenital astigmatism or acquired myopia when there is relative lack of demand for accommodation. This may also be seen in cases of high hypermetropia and myopic astigmatism.

Similarly debility from any cause has a tendency by weakening convergence to induce exophoria temporarily as in overwork, emotional situations, and chronic debilitating disease, etc.

Neurogenic Heterophoria

Faulty innervational control of the eyes such as irregular excitation of lower cortical centres, disturbances of the proprioceptive connections of the oculomotor apparatus and incoordination of the higher centres, etc. may account for certain cases of heterophia. Physical or mental fatigue as also ill health may lessen control over the coordination of the eyes so that deviations (which otherwise would have been constantly compensated) become apparent.

The power of fusion has a considerable etiological bearing on heterophoria. When it is well developed, a great fusional amplitude allows even larger deviations to remain latent and symptom-free. When it is poorly developed, a condition of binocular instability results which gives rise to symptoms. And fusion is constantly breaking with the onset of fatigue or with increased difficulties offered by intermittent changes in the distance or direction of the fixation point.

Anatomical anomalies cause essential or static heterophoria, whereas the one of accommodative origin leads to symptomatic heterophoria. This accommodative one is amenable to treatment by refractive correction (if any), orthoptic exercises or symptomatic treatment. Static heterophoria on the other hand is amenable to operative correction only.

Diagnosis and Measurement: A careful and detailed history is the first essential requisite in diagnosis and management of cases of heterophoria. This should include patients' complaints, the precise nature of his work and hobbies, previous history of ocular trouble, wearing of glasses and any other treatment. Routine eye examination as also examination for general medical status are then carried out. Refraction should be carefully estimated using cycloplegia. Thereafter, necessary glasses are prescribed. Many a times correction of the refractive error (by reducing the muscular imbalance) is all that may be necessary to relieve the symptoms of heterophoria. (Figs 9.1 to 9.6).

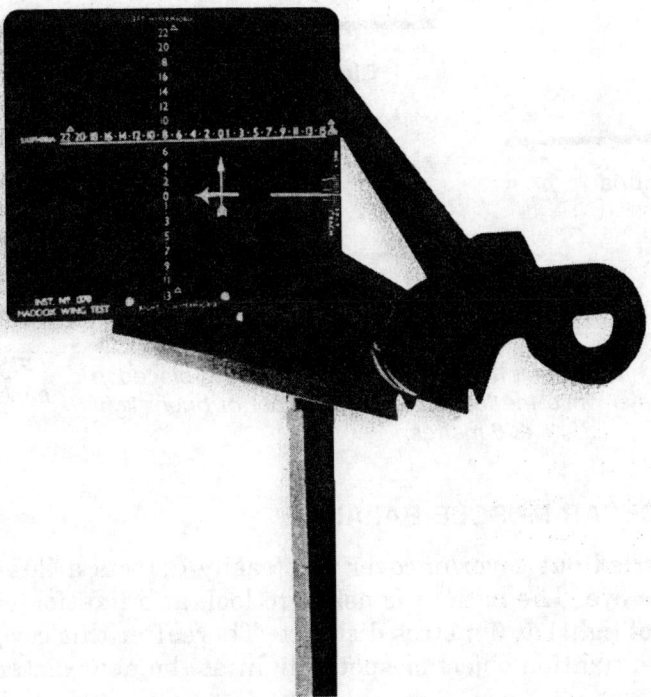

Fig. 9.1: *Maddox wing.*

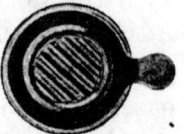

Fig. 9.2:   Maddox rod.

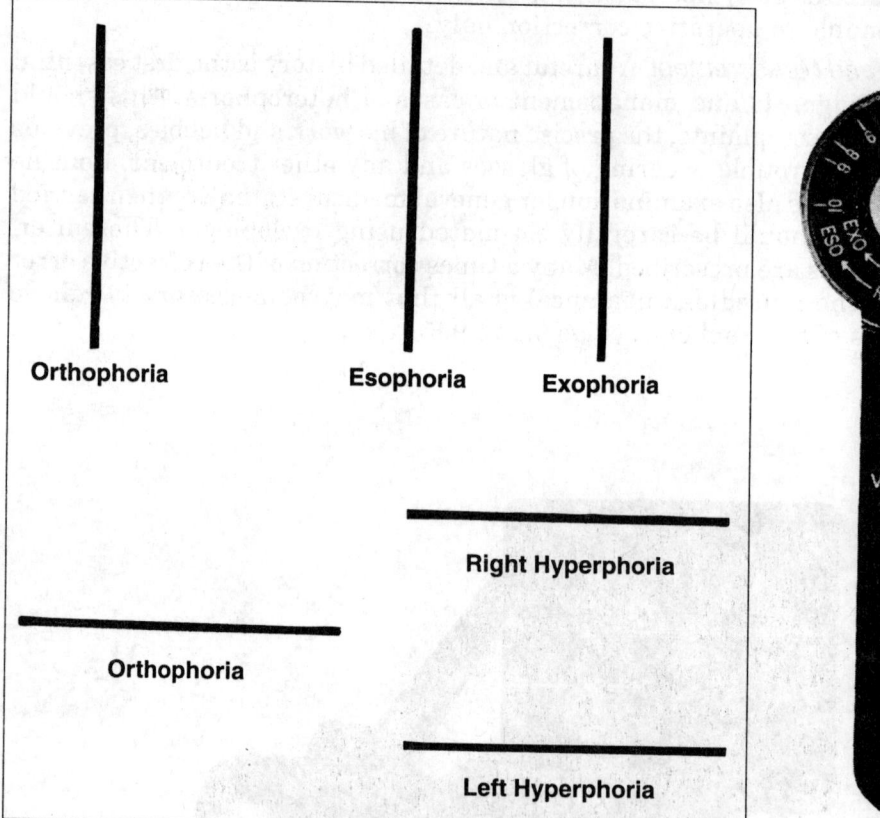

Orthophoria   Esophoria   Exophoria

Right Hyperphoria

Orthophoria

Left Hyperphoria

Fig. 9.3:   Maddox rod test for heterophoria. Maddox rod is placed in front of the right eye while the left eye sees the spot of bright light at 6 metres.

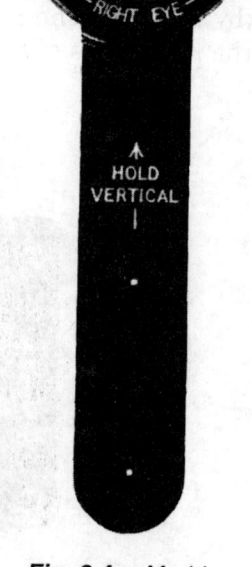

Fig. 9.4:   Maddox hand frame uniocular.

EXTRINSIC OCULAR MUSCLE BALANCE

A carefully carried out cover/uncover test easily detects a latent or manifest deviation of the eye. The patient is asked to look at a fixation object (which is usually a spot of light) at 6 metres distance. Thereafter this cover/uncover test is repeated for a fixation object or spot of light at the near distance of 33 cm.

The test is carried out first with the patient wearing his corrective glasses (if any) and then without the glasses.

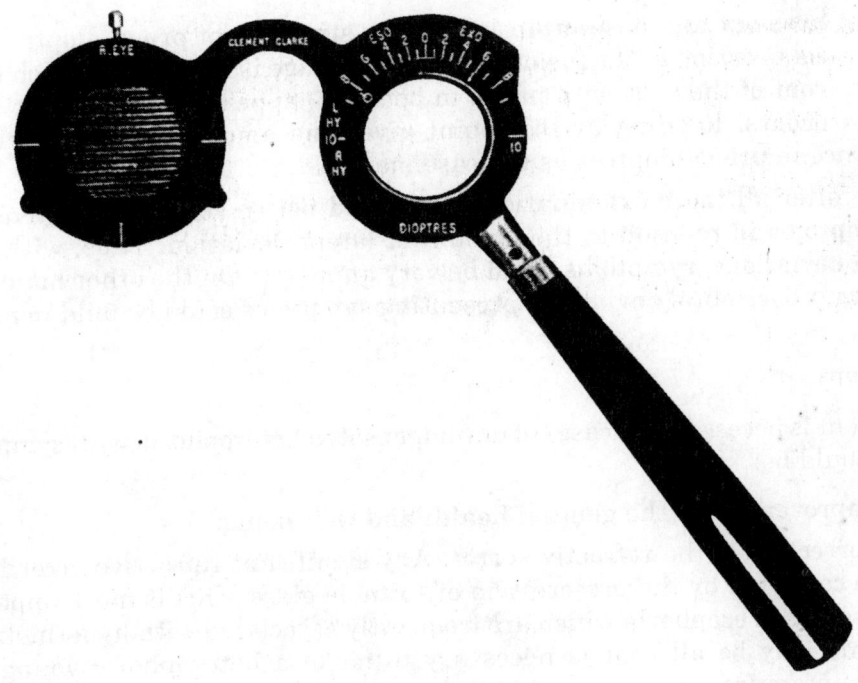

Fig. 9.5: *Maddox hand frame. They measure the heterophoric deviation in prism of dioptre.*

At 33 cm (near fixation distance) use is made of Maddox-wing to detect the presence and amount of latent deviation eso-, exo-, hyper- or hypophoria.

A Maddox-rod is used for the 6 metre distance cover test to detect and measure the amount of latent deviation. A Maddox tangent scale (Fig. 9.6) helps.

Using a Maddox-hand frame, the amount of latent deviation or heterophoria is easily measured in prism-dioptres.

Assessment of the State of Binocular Vision

This is necessary for symptoms of heterophoria also depend on the state of binocular single vision. A full fusional reserve indicates a well-compensated heterophoria which would not be expected to produce symptoms.

Such an assessment is carried out on a major amblyoscope (*see* Fig. 7.2).

Simultaneous macular perception (SMP), fusional-reserve or range of fusion and the degree of stereoscopic vision all these three have to be assessed. The range of fusion (or fusional-reserve) normally should be 30° to 35° degree of convergence (adduction), 5° to 8° degree of divergence (abduction) and 3° to 4° degree of vertical vergence as measured from 0 degree on a major-amblyoscope. In most cases of symptom-producing heterophoria, the range of fusion is defective.

Prism base-out and base-in, in increasing strength (of prism dioptre) could also be used to estimate the fusional reserve. A stage is reached at which letters (kept in front of the eyes with prism in between) appear blurred before actual diplopia occurs. Reading at this point gives the amount of convergence or divergence in prism dioptres as the case may be.

Even after all these examinations, one could not be sure of the intensity of the symptoms in relation to the amount of latent-deviation. Thus, with small vertical deviations, symptoms could be very annoying. On the other hand, even with larger horizontal deviations presenting symptoms could be mild in nature.

Treatment

Treatment is necessary for cases of uncompensated heterophoria with symptoms. These could be:

i. Improvement of the general health and well-being.

ii. Correction of the refractive error: Any significant refractive error has to be corrected by the prescription of suitable glass. This is more important in cases of esophoria which are frequently associated with hypermetropia. This may be all that is necessary to make a heterophoric young man symptom-free.

Prisms

Prisms may be necessary to relieve symptoms in certain cases of esophoria, exophoria and hypo- or hyperphoria. Actually prisms are valuable for orthoptic exercise. Convergence could be toned up by use of base out prisms, thus relieving symptoms in these cases of esophoria.

As a part of treatment, prescribing prisms (incorporated in the correcting glass by altering the position of the optical centre of the glass) is sometimes necessary, when orthoptic treatment fails to relieve symptoms and where operation is contraindicated as in the case of an elderly patient and in those suffering from heterophoria of the unstable and progressive nature. While prescribing prisms, it should be incorporated in both the glasses right and left, i.e. half of the total dioptric value of the prism in each glass. The strength of the prism should not exceed 6 Δ in each lens (glass).

Orthoptic Treatment

The essence of orthoptic treatment is to teach adequate and effortless convergence and divergence, thereby improving binocular function. While improving the convergence, there may be a temporary increase in the amount of esophoria but, as convergence becomes increasingly effortless, esophoria tends to decrease. With poor convergence one has to make extra effort to maintain binocular single vision when viewing near objects. This causes sustained contraction of the medial rectus muscle giving rise to esophoria and symptoms of eye-strain.

A comfortable harmony between accommodation and convergence is necessary for symptom-free vision. To achieve this, accommodation has to be relaxed while convergence is being exercised on an amblyoscope. In cases of exophoria, exercise to increase fusional convergence and relax divergence are very useful to make the patient symptom-free.

To begin with, orthoptic treatment has to be given on a major amblyoscope or synoptophore.

A normal healthy adult should achieve some 35° to 45° degree of convergence on a symptophore. A child or an elderly presbyope would have convergence less than this amount. One way of improving convergence is by the use of concave lens of 3 to 6 dioptre placed in the lens holder of the synoptophore. This causes more accommodation to be exercised which in turn stimulates convergence. Sometimes this may cause accommodative spasm. Hence the use of SMP and fusion slides is more useful in improving the convergence.

Normal-divergence range is − 3° to − 6° degree. It is advisable to give divergence exercise after practicing convergence. This induces relaxation.

After a few sessions on synoptophore, home-exercise is equally necessary for a long period of symptom-free state of heterophoris.

1. Teaching the patient to appreciate physiological diplopia both for near and distance using pencil or some small liner object is necessary (Fig. 9.6). It must be appreciated that this is an arduous task causing initially a lot of discomfort and eye-strain and thus many a times given up. But persistence brings its rewards.
2. Once physiological diplopia is appreciated, the next exercise is to teach convergence to a near point using the same pencil or the small linear object. The pencil should be held at a distance of twelve to eighteen inches from the patient's eye and is then moved slowly nearer to the nose till it is seen to be double. This should be repeated about a dozen times, the patient trying to keep the pencil appear single for a longer period at each attempt.

A number of suitable instruments like stereograms, diploscopes, stereoscopes, etc. are available for home exercise but they all need the help and guidance of a trained orthoptist.

Surgery

In a few obstinate cases and where orthoptic exercises are not feasible, surgical interference is necessary to make heterophoria symptom-free. This is particularly so when dealing with vertical phoria — hyper- or hypophoria. The surgical details are more or less the same as in cases of heterotropia (manifest strabismus).

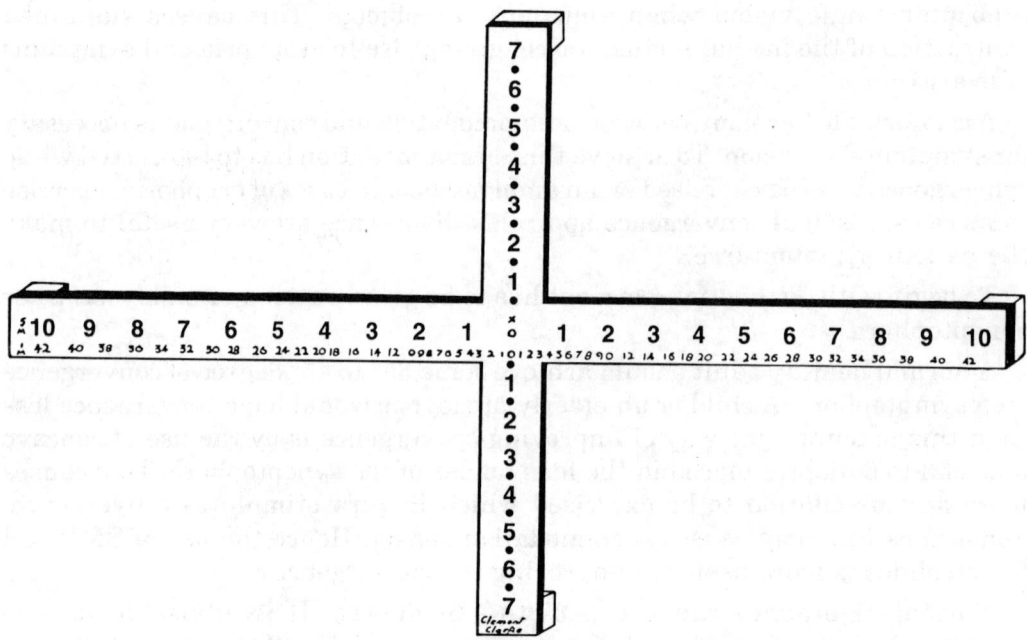

Fig. 9.6: *Maddox tangent scale to measure the deviation at 6 metres.*

Surgical correction is particularly applicable in cases of static heterophoria where symptoms develop and which do not respond to treatment (as described above) including prescription of prisms incorporated in the glass.

Esophoria

Esophoria is more common than exophoria. It is associated with less distressing symptoms but is more difficult to treat. As stated earlier convergence-excess type of esophoria is more common.

Etiologically an increased convergence innervation associated with increased accommodation consequent on a hypermetropic refractive error is the main factor. Patients with opacities in ocular media have to unduly strain their accommodation for increased clarity of vision and in so doing they inadvertently use more of convergence and, thus get symptoms of eye-strain or asthenopia.

Static anatomical conditions in the orbit play a relatively minor role. Esophoria is more common in young neurotic type of individuals.

Headache, blurring of vision and undue ocular-fatigue, particularly after reading or near work, constitute the main symptoms. Some times discomfort accompanies the use of the eyes at all distances. Mental irritation and psychological disturbance may follow in the neurotic type of individuals. A manifest dissociation causing intermittent diplopia may be seen where fusion-power is no longer able to provide the requisite binocularity.

A full correction of any refractive error is the first line of treatment. Refraction should be determined under a cycloplegic. When full correction is not tolerated, distance may be undercorrected for clarity and comfort but for near vision and work, full correction should be prescribed.

In orthoptic exercise the use of relieving prisms, base out is sometimes of value. In some cases where despite orthoptic exercise symptoms are not relieved and surgery is not feasible prism base out may be incorporated in the glass used by the patients (Fig. 9.7).

Surgical relief is effective in cases of essential esophoria and not for accommodational-convergence or innervational type of cases.

The general health and psychological upsetting factors have to be carefully analysed and taken care of whenever and wherever necessary.

Exophoria

Herein, there is a tendency for the eyes to diverge which is held in check by fusional impulses. It is more common in advancing age and when the general health is poor.

Disturbance of accommodation–convergence ratio plays a minor role in the etiology. An uncorrected myope does not exercise his accommodation fully and this may lead to a latent divergence developing in adult life.

A neurogenic etiology in the shape of disturbance of the central innervation mechanism controlling convergence and divergence is rare.

Symptoms Headaches, blurring of vision and fatigue are normally (usually) more marked during close work which may become impossible to bear.

Failure of fusion may cause intermittent diplopia. Of all heterophorias, treatment of exophoria is more satisfactory.

Refractive error (hypermetropia, astigmatism or presbyonia) has to be corrected. Cases of astigmatism and myopia have to be fully corrected while hypermetropia and presbyopia need undercorrection. This encourages accommodation which in turn leads to convergence being exercised.

Orthoptic exercises to increase fusional convergence and relax divergence are very useful in cases of exophoria.

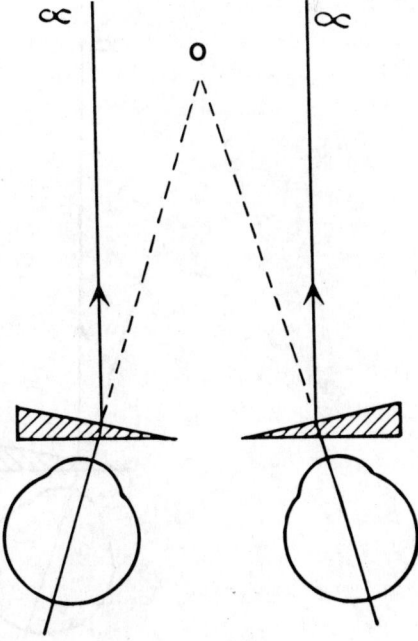

Fig. 9.7: *Esophoria correction by prism base out.*

Relieving prisms base-in (Fig. 9.8) are of considerable value, particularly for near work, and may be necessary in some cases of static nature to relieve symptoms. This may be particularly necessary in those where operative interference is not feasible.

Cyclophoria

A tendency for one eye to wheel-rotate relative to the other is cyclophoria. The vertical axis of cornea or upper end of vertical meridian tends to deviate inwards or outwards incylophoria or excyclophoria respectively.

Uncorrected oblique astigmation is an important cause of cyclophoria. The amount of cyclophoria that can be overcome without symptoms arising varies with individuals. The symptoms are headache, nausea and even vomiting.

Head-tilting (generally associated with ocular muscle palsy) may also be present in cyclophoria. It is probably produced as much in the interest of correcting the leaning of the image as of raising or lowering the false image.

Treatment

Correction of the refractive error may be all that is necessary for the relief of symptoms.

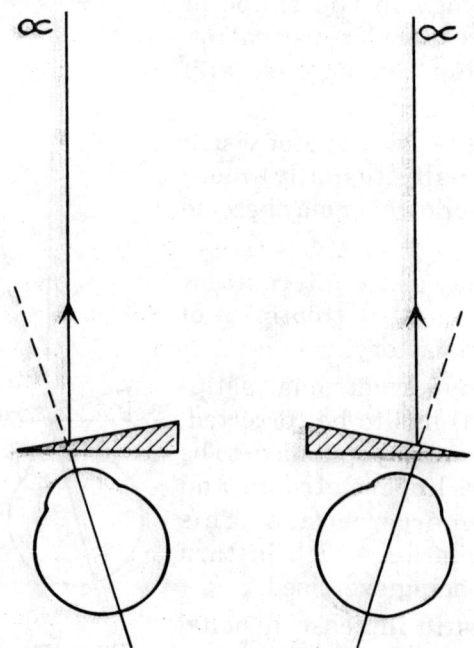

Fig. 9.8: *Exophoria correction by prism base in.*

Orthoptic exercise on a synoptophore is necessary in some cases. The muscles concerned in cyclophoria are the two oblique the superior and inferior oblique. Superior oblique causes intortion while inferior oblique leads to extortion. Hence, for excyclophoria due to overaction of inferior oblique, this muscle needs weakening. And in those where excyclophoria is from insufficiency of superior oblique, this muscle has to be strengthened Vice versa is true for incyclophoria from weakness of inferior oblique or from overaction of superior oblique. Necessary surgical procedure may have to be taken recourse to.

REFERENCES

1. Adler F. H: Pathological physiology of convergent strabismus: Motor aspect of the non-accommodational type. *Arch. Ophthalmol*. 33: 352, 1945.
2. Chavasse F. B.: *Worth's Squint or the Binocular Reflexes and the Treatment of Strabismus*, 7th edn. Philadelphia, P. Blackiston's Son & Co, 1939.
3. Dufier J. L., Briard M. L., Bonaiti C., Frezal J. and Laurex H.: Inheritance in the etiology of congenital squint. *Ophthalmologica* 179: 225, 1979.
4. Friedrich D. and de Decker W.: Prospective study of the development of strabismus during the first six months of life, in Lenk-Schafer M. (Editor) *Trans. Sixth International Orthoptic Congress*, Harrogate, 1987, p. 21.
5. Maumenee I. H., Alston A. Mets M. B. et al: Inheritance of congenital esotropia. *Trans. Am. Ophthalmol*. Soc. 84: 85, 1985.
6. Noorden G. K. Von: Current concepts of infantile esotropia: The William Bowman Lecture. *Eye*, 2 : 243, 1988.
7. Nordlow N. Age distribution at the onset of esotropia. *Br. J. Ophthalmol*., 37: 593, 1953.
8. Pratt-Johnson J. A.: Central disruption of fusional amplitude. *Br. J. Ophthalmol*., 57: 347, 1973.
9. Rohatgi J. N.: Intermittent Exotropia. *Proc. 44th All India Ophthalmol. Conference*, Kanpur, India, 1986.
10. Scholossman A. and Priestlay B.S.: Role of hereditary in etiology and treatment of strabismus. *Arch. Ophthalmol*., 47 : 1, 1952.
11. Stanworth A: Defects of ocular movement and fusion after head injury. *Br. J. Ophthalmol*., 58: 266, 1974.
12. Tychsen L., Hurtig R. R. and Scott W. E: Pursuit is impaired but the vestibulo-ocular reflex is normal in infantile strabismus. *Arch. Ophthalmol*., 103, 506, 1985.
13. Tychsen L. and Lisberger S. L.: Visual motion processing for the initiation of smooth pursuit eye movement in humans *J. Neurophysiol*., 56 : 953, 1986.
14. Worth C.: *Squint: Its Causes, Pathology and Treatment*, 6th edn. London, Bailliere Tindall & Cox, 1929.

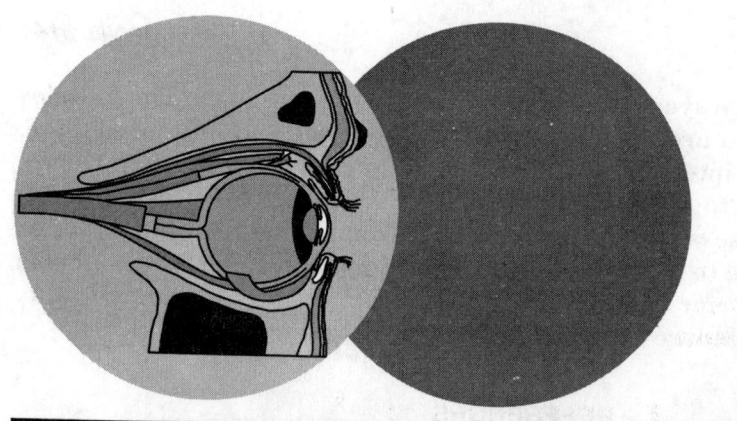

Concomitant Squint
Heterotropia

A concomitant squint is a deviation of the eyes, where the deviation remains the same in all directions of the gaze. Such cases could be broadly divided etiologically into two types—Primary (the great majority) and the secondary (which has a peripheral muscular basis — insufficiency or paresis). The primary type is centrally initiated.

Clinically cases of concomitant strabismus could be (1) convergent or esotropia, (2) divergent or exotropia, and (3) a few cases of hypo-/hypertropia. These latter ones are mostly associated with vertical-muscle imbalance and are considered as a group of cyclo-vertical deviation. Hence, they are not being discussed in this chapter.

CONCOMITANT CONVERGENT STRABISMUS (ESOTROPIA)

The great majority of strabismus cases belong to this group. They have been variously classified, partly on the basis of etiological factors and partly on the basis of clinical findings. A working classification as given in Von Noorden: "*Binocular Vision and Ocular Motility*, 4th edn, 1990, could be modified as follows.

    I. *Accommodational*
        a. Fully accommodative
           (i) Normal AC/A ratio.

(ii) High AC/A ratio — Accommodative convergence excess type of esotropia.
    b. Partly accommodative.

II. *Non-Accommodative*
    a. Infantile esotropia.
    b. Acquired esotropia   i. Basic type
                             ii. Convergence-excess type
                             iii. Esotropia in myopia.
    c. Microtropia.

III. *Secondary esodeviation and consecutive esotropia*

Accommodative-concomitant convergent strabismus is a type of concomitant squint in which the convergent deviation of the eye varies in degree or dioptre according to the amount of accommodation exerted.

In the fully accommodative type with normal Ac/A ratio, the wearing of glasses (to correct the hypermetropia) eliminates the deviation, so that there is good binocular vision along with good visual acuity. And in the absence of the glass, there is usually a manifest deviation (Fig. 10.1).

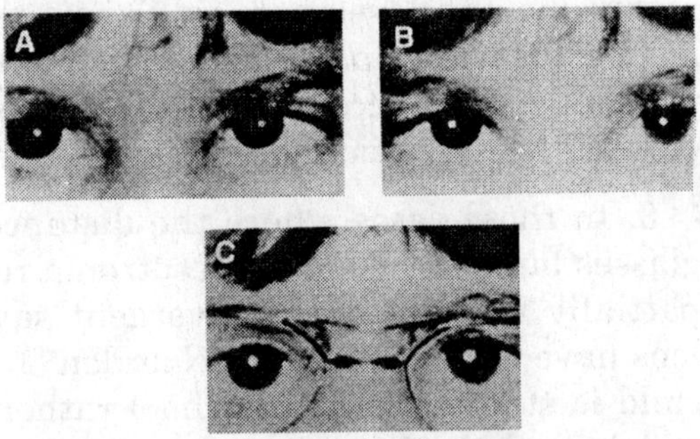

Two etiological components, uncorrected hypermetropia and insufficient fusional divergence/or excessive convergence, contribute to this type of deviation.

Fig. 10.1: *A case of left convergent squint — fully accommodative in nature using glass. Note that deviation is corrected with glass so long it is being used.*

An uncorrected hypermetrope uses excessive accommodation to clearly see an object both at distance and at near fixation. This brings into play the synergic convergence and thus, excessive amount of convergence is used. To counteract this excessive convergence, if the amplitude of fusional divergence is adequate, the deviation may remain as esophoria. But when the fusional divergence is inadequate, the esodeviation becomes manifest convergent. Or esotropia.

The onset of accommodative-esotropia is classically between 2 and 3 years of age, when the awakening intelligence of children begins to demand clarity of near objects and thus, the use of accommodative-convergence faculty. However, cases of accommodative-strabismus have been reported in children of one year of age or even earlier.

The ocular deviation is uniocular and variable in amount (degree or prism dioptre), being greater at near fixation than at distance-fixation. The deviation may pass through the stage of intermittency before becoming constant. In this stage, the child gets asthenopic symptoms. He complains of intermittent diplopia and may like to close one eye when doing near work.

Treatment and Management

Treatment and management of these cases comprise the following.

1. Full correction of the hypermetropic refractive error as determined by cycloplegic refraction is the first step. If the deviation is not fully controlled, it may be advisable to repeat the refraction under cycloplegia, after, the glasses have been worn for a few months. If, there, is any likelihood that the first test failed to unmask the full extent of the hypermetropia - this is all the more necessary.

2. Correct assessment of visual acuity in the deviating eye with glasses is necessary. And when the visual acuity is not fully corrected with glasses or amblyopia has developed, amblyopia therapy of occluding the sound eye has to be taken recourse to. However, it is unusual to find a marked degree of amblyopia in cases of fully accommodative strabismus, because of the comparatively late onset of the deviation and, the fact, that it is often intermittent in character.

3. In those cases where the distance-deviation is reduced or eliminated by glasses but some degree of esotropia remains at near fixation (cases of fully or partially accommodate convergent squint), use of a weaker miotic or bifocal lens have to be thought of (Noorden[20]) one would prefer a bifocal lens when the child is studying or/is at school rather than using a miotic. But authors vary widely in their choice based on personal experience of treating such cases.

4. *Use of orthoptic treatment* In all types of accommodative convergent squint cases, the purpose of orthoptic treatment or exercise is (Lyle)[16].

  a. To overcome suppression, particularly at the convergent angle of deviation,
  b. To treat the patient-relaxation of accommodation with consequent relaxation of convergence.
  c. To teach dissociation of accommodation and convergence that is, to dissociate accommodation from that part of convergence which is variable, and
  d. To ensure that the patient develops good binocular convergence.

5. Recourse to surgery, when the deviation is large and not fully corrected by use of glasses.

6. Depending on the age of the child and his cooperation (a child may be too young to cooperate for orthoptic exercises) pre- and or post-operative orthoptic exercises are given or suggested to ensure a comfortable binocular vision in all circumstances so that the patient has a good range of fusion with full binocular convergence.

Most children with refractive accommodative esotropia have an excellent outcome in terms of visual acuity and binocular single vision. "Current management strategies for this condition result in a marked reduction in the prevalence of amblyopia compared with the prevalence at presentation. The degree of hypertropia, however, remains unchanged with poor prospect for discontinuing glass wear" Alan Mulvihill et al[18].

Accommodative Esotropia with Convergence Excess (or with High AC/A Ratio)

While in a fully accommodative convergent squint AC/A ratio is normal or nearly normal, one comes across children with an abnormally high AC/A ratio (Parks, 1958)[22]. Examination reveals esotropia (convergence) which is greater at near fixation than at distance fixation. An analysis of refractive error indicates a moderate degree of hypermetropia and sometimes emmetropia or myopia. In these cases, it is presumed that there is an abnormal synkinesis between accommodation and accommodative convergence (AC) so that an effort of accommodation elicits an abnormally high accommodative convergence reflex. Even with the refractive error fully corrected, there is a significant esodeviation at near fixation.

Treatment

The convergent deviation at near fixation may be overcome by the temporary use of additional convex spherical lenses for near vision where a correction for hypermetropia is already being worn. Prescribing a bifocal-glass or clip-on lenses to be worn over the patients own glass while reading serves the purpose. But then a prolonged use of bifocals is not desirable. It may prevent the development of normal accommodation. Partial occlusion and orthoptic exercises are necessary to improve accommodation and teach development of fusional divergence amplitude. Some prefer to use miotics in such cases to control the deviation.

Partially Accommodative Esotropia (Convergent Strabismus)

In a number of children with convergent squint (Fig. 10.2), despite full correction of the hypermetropic refractive error, prescription of a bifocal lens and or use of miotics, a residual esodeviation or convergence may exist. Though the visual axes are convergent in all circumstances, the deviation increases when accommodation is exerted and when the hypermetropic correction is removed or not used. Such cases may be of the following two types -

a. The esotropia or convergence has been congenital/early infantile or even paretic and as the child grows older an accommodative element becomes superimposed and increases the deviation.

b. These cases may have been of the fully accommodative type, but due to lack of suitable treatment, got decompensated and became cases of manifest deviation all the time.

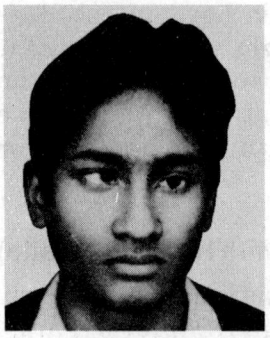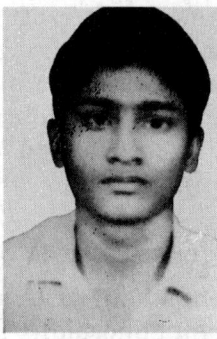

Fig. 10.2: *A case of right convergent squint — partially accommodative in type before operation. After operation the eyes looked straight.*

Treatment[13] Warranted by the size of the angle of deviation, surgery may have to be performed to align the eyes and glasses would continue to be used after surgery.

Keenan and Willshaw (1993)[12] writing about the outcome of strabismus surgery in childhood esotropia mention that a favourable outcome with evidence of binocular single vision is the expected outcome in the majority of children with partially accommodative esotropia. The surgical strategy should aim for a final post-operative alignment within + 10 Δ dioptres of straight or within + 20 Δ diopters of straight if there was evidence of binocular single vision.

NON-ACCOMMODATIONAL CONVERGENT DEVIATION

Essential-Infantile Esotropia

It is unilateral convergent strabismus and in some cases with a tendency to alternate.

Esotropia with an onset at birth or during infancy may result from many different causes. But when we talk of congenital esotropia (now better known as essential infantile esotropia), it is a specific entity with an onset between birth and 6 months of age and whose etiology is essentially unknown. The clinical features (Noorden)[19, 21] are as follows:

i. Onset of deviation before 6 months of the age.

ii. A large angle of deviation generally more than 15⁰ or 30 (prism-dioptre).

iii. The angle of deviation is stable and the same both for distance and near-fixation and hence a normal Ac/A ratio.

iv. Initially the deviation may be alternating in nature — Essential alternating convergent squint.

v. Varying refractive error — generally low-grade hypermetropia (Costenbader[4]).

vi. Most children with infantile esotropia exhibit apparent defective abduction and excessive adduction or both. Due to lack of this movement chavasse[3] called it "habitual inhibition of abduction".

vii. Amblyopia: It is commonly associated with infantile esotropia.

viii. Poor binocular single vision or potential for developing BSV is poor.

ix. Normal central nervous system.

x. Latent or manifest nystagmus.

xi. Associated vertical deviation — primary overaction of inferior oblique and dissociated vertical deviations are common.

xii. The head and face may appear to be tilted towards the shoulder of the fixing eye in some cases.

The esodeviation or convergence has a tendency to decrease with passage of time and this justifies conservatism with regard to early surgical treatment of these children.

Defective abduction in one or both eyes suggests the possibility of paresis of one or both lateral rectus muscle. However, a slight defect of abduction which Chavasse[3] described as "habitual inhibition of abduction" may be the result of lack of movement in this direction, for in a convergent squint of long standing a contracture of the medial rectus muscle may cause an apparent weakness of the direct antagonist (lateral rectus muscle).

Treatment: The treatment for infantile-esotropia is surgical alignment of the eye. Any hypermetropia has to be carefully assessed and suitable glass prescribed. When amblyopia exists occlusion of the sound eye should be instituted before surgery.

Even with careful and frequent follow up by experienced clinicians a number of children with infantile exotropia develop a significant degree of amblyopia after surgical alignment whereas if these children remain untreated, the risk of strabismic amblyopia is much lower.

"Early alignment will produce some degree of binocular single vision and stability but also some risk of amblyopia. But with a delaying surgery until the patient is a visual adult, there is lesser degree of binocular single vision but a smaller risk of amblyopia" (Tony Murray, 1993)[17].

Noorden[19] (1990) emphasises that any child whose eyes are not aligned by three months of age, should be given a complete ophthalmic examination even though treatment may not be possible or necessary on the first visit.

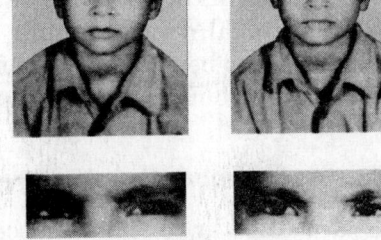

Alternating Concomitant Squint

Congenital Alternating Squint

Essential alternating squint (Fig. 10.3) or essential alternators is usually of early onset, rather the infant is born with squint. The deviation at birth may not be obvious enough to attract attention. It tends, however, to increase as the infant begins to grow. The

Fig. 10.3: *A case of alternating convergent squint.*

essential alternators are supposed to be due to defective or poor or non-development of fusion faculty. In some of them, however, normal binocular single vision has developed when an accurate operative correction was done at an early age to allow the binocular reflexes to become established.

Innervational

In cases of acquired myopia of 5 to 6 dioptre about the age of puberty, some children show a tendency for squint. Such a deviation is variable in amount 15^0 to 20^0 and tends to be alternating rather than uniocular-good vision being retained-in each eye. A disuse of accommodation in these myopes with a consequential weakness of convergence makes up the typical clinical picture of convergence-insufficiency progressing to manifest divergent squint, alternating more than uniocular.

The child uses each eye indiscriminately or sometimes at will because the vision and refractive-error in the eyes are more or less equal. They occur preferentially in hypermetropes and develop typically around the age of 3 years or more since older the child, the more difficult is the development of uniocular inhibition. They may have an element of rudimentary binocular single vision (primary type of alternating squint).

The main clinical features of an alternating squint are: Noorden[21], Duke-Elder[6], Rohatgi[23].

   i.   Early onset of squint or its presence from birth.
  ii.   A large angle of deviation generally 20^0 or more.
 iii.   More or less equal visual acuity in each eye.
  iv.   No significant refractive error or equal degree of ammetropia.
   v.   Free alternation.
  vi.   Absence of development of amblyopia.
 vii.   Visual comfort by facultative-suppression.

Treatment: It is mainly operative-straightening of the eyes in one or two sittings. And the earlier it is done, the better is the result. At least, the cosmetic blemish is gone and this helps in the development of a proper psyche in the child. Besides, early surgical straightening of the eye followed by postoperative orthoptic exercises has been shown to help some children develop some form of binocular vision even though it may be anomalous.

Non-Accommodative Acquired Esotropia

Esodeviation or concomitant convergent squints with onset after six (6) months of age with little or no accommodative component are being discussed in this group (Fig. 10.4). They may be of (1) basic type, (2) convergent excess type, or (3) esotropia in myopia.

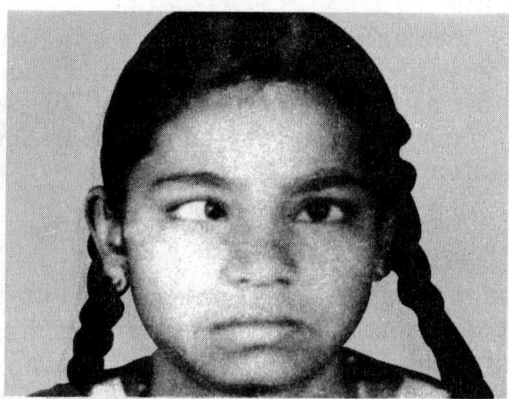

Fig. 10.4: *Non–accommodative left convergent squint in a 10-year old girl.*

The Basic Type

Cases of concomitant convergent squint with onset after 6 months of age but limited to childhood with the following clinical features of (i) Insignificant refractive error, (ii) no accommodational factor, (iii) deviation for Distance and near-fixation more or less equal in degree, and (iv) with no ocular movement restriction.

They are included in the basic type of non-accommodative acquired esotropia. Parents frequently associate the onset of deviation or squint with illness or injury. The vision in the squinting eye is less than in the normal eye but there is no significant refractive error. Hence, such children do not respond to the use of glasses. Some ophthalmologists, however, like to prescribe the glass in these cases on the basis of physiological hypermetropia in this age group which may vary from + 3.00 Dsph to + 1.00 Dsph (on retinoscopy).

An attempt has to be made to treat the amblyopia by occlusion of the sound eye. And this is followed by surgical correction of the deviation. Almost two-thirds of these children (with basic type of non-accommodative esotropia) may be expected to obtain a favourable outcome and with less than half developing evidence of binocular single vision. This result might be improved by increasing the amount of surgery (Keenan and Willshaw, 1993)[12]. These authors suggest conjunctival recession, bimedial recession of 7 mm and three muscle surgery (which should be considered for a pre-operative squint angle of 45 Δ dioptres or larger). Occlusion for amblyopia may also be continued after surgical correction of the deviation. This would help in improving BSV (fusion aspect of it).

The Non-Accommodative Convergence—Excess Type of Esotropia

Cases of concomitant convergent squint manifesting in children between 2 and 3 years of age, with small angle convergence at distant fixation and a larger esotropia (20 to 40⁰) at near-fixation and with no accommodative component pose an etiological problem. Some of these children are hypermetropic and some are emmetropic. They have excessive convergence other than accommodative, perhaps from tonic innervation. And hence are referred to as convergence excess type of esotropia. As far as treatment is concerned, surgery is the choice for prescription of glasses (bifocal) and use of miotic drops are found to be ineffective in controlling the deviation for near fixation.

Esotropia in Myopia

In moderate congenital myopia, the young child does not use his accommodation. He can see clearly at near distance using his convergence as the far point of clear vision is near at hand. Vision in distance is blurred so that no effort is made to avoid diplopia beyond the far point. Binocularity for distance is usually absent with dense suppression. The position of excessive convergence purposively adopted for near vision is, therefore, retained for all distances and becomes consolidated. There is a comfortable binocular vision for near fixation and hence, no diplopia.

In grown-up children and young adults (20 to 40 years of age) with myopia and who have not been corrected or are undercorrected by glasses — a similar convergent squint may occur after binocularity has been established (in acquired myopia). Constant reliance on near vision and neglect of objects in distance over a period of years, leads to a functional deficiency of divergence resulting in the appearance of periodic squint.

In very young children with myopia and convergent squint as described above, treatment involves the constant use of full corrective glasses. In this way, convergence is discouraged, accommodation stimulated and a normal accommodation-convergence relationship is built up which can be sustained by orthoptic exercises (as soon as the child is capable for these exercises) and supplemented by surgical correction, when otherwise unsuccessful. In young adults and grown up children with acquired myopia and convergent squint- similarly the refractive error has to be corrected and surgical correction of the deviation undertaken.

Microtropia

Lang[14] (1966) introduced the term micro strabismus and microtropia to describe a uniocular small angle heterotropia of less than 5° associated with harmonius abnormal retinal correspondence, mild amblyopia and partial stereopsis. According to him microtropia occurs in 2 forms, viz. (a) primary and (b) secondary. The secondary form of microtropia is seen more often after surgical correction of an essential infantile esotropia. The primary one remains constant during life or the angle of heterotropia may increase.

In every case of microtropia, eccentric-fixation and some degree of amblyopia are present in one eye. The size of this ultra-small tropia equals the distance in the amblyopic eye between the fovea and the area used for eccentric-fixation (called pseudo-fovea). Because of a unique sensory adaptation, the eccentric area of the deviating eye is used both for binocular as well as monocular vision and thus, no refixation movement on cover test is required by the amblyopic eye when the foveally fixing eye is covered. The cover-test for tropia, the cover-uncover test for phoria and the alternate cover-test to demonstrate the maximum deviation have to be carried out meticulously and repeatedly before diagnosing a case of microtropia.

A 4-dioptre-prism placed over the foveally fixing eye will elicit a tropia because of the small central scotoma in the eccentrically fixing amblyopic eye.

Bifoveal Correspondence Test

This test and the Bagolini striated glass-test demonstrate the harmonious adaptation between the fovea of the sound eye and eccentrically fixing area of amblyopic eye. According to Helveston and Noorden (1967)[9] it is reasonable to assume that even small degree of anisometropia, if left uncorrected in early childhood, may lead to the establishment of a scotoma, anisometropic amblyopia and finally to microstrabismus. Uncorrected anisometropia seems to be the principal cause of the central scotoma.

Esotropia Secondary Convergent Squint

Organic ocular conditions that affect the visual acuity in one eye (reducing the vision in that eye substantially) may cause a unilateral convergent squint in that eye. And as such a routine examination of the eye under a mydriatic is a must in all cases of strabismus.

Cases of unilateral corneal leucoma (specially the ones in centre of cornea and dense in intensity) congenital or traumatic unilateral cataract, a patient of chorio retinal inflammation involving the macular area, optic atrophy (all unilateral) produce convergent squint in the affected eye. All these pathologies present a severe obstacle to sensory-fusion or may abolish the fusion-mechanism altogether.

Depending on the age of the child (at the time of visual acuity decrease), esotropia or exotopia may develop in that eye. In children below the age of 5-6 years, these factors generally produce a convergent squint and in those above the ages of 8-9 years, the very same factors are likely to produce a divergent deviation in that eye.

Treatment is naturally that of the cause. Once the causative factor is no longer active or has been treated, operation is indicated for squint on cosmetic grounds. Full binocular vision is obviously unattainable in these cases.

Secondary Consecutive Convergent Squint

Theoretically a convergent squint may result from surgical overcorrection of a divergent squint. But it is not commonly seen. In some of these, a spontaneous decrease of convergence is described, while in others a surgical correction of the overcorrected divergent eye may become necessary.

Convergent squint associated with vertical deviations and following convergent or long standing ocular palsy need some discussion.

With Associated Vertical Deviations

An overaction of the inferior oblique muscle is seen quite often in children with convergent squint giving a vertical component to the esodeviation. In the constant adducted position of the eye, oblique muscles come into play and because the inferior oblique is mechanically superior to superior oblique muscle, in this adducted position the eyes goes up as a result of inferior oblique overaction.

After the necessary surgery on horizontal muscle in such cases, the overaction of the inferior oblique disappears. This confirms, that the overaction of the inferior oblique muscle is secondary to the horizontal convergent deviation.

That A and V syndrome, in which the eso- and exo-deviation vary with the eye in up and down position are examples of associated vertical deviations based or superimposed on primary concomitant deviation and are being considered separately.

(b) In long standing cases of ocular muscles palsy, in which little or no recovery of the paralysed muscle has occurred, as well as in cases of ocular palsy of congenital origin, changes occur in the muscles of the affected eye as also in the muscles of the unaffected eye. These are an overaction of the ipsilateral antagonist, contraction of the contra-lateral synergist and inhibitional palsy of the contralateral antagonist. The result of these changes is that the deviation gradually tends to assume the characteristics of concomitance. In the case of paresis of a horizontally acting muscle, concomitance may eventually occur in all positions of the gaze whereas in the case of a vertically acting muscle, concomitance usually occurs in dextro- or laevo-version only depending on the muscle at fault.

Prism-Adaptation

The preoperative use of prisms in an acquired esotopia to determine the maximum angle of strabismus and to estimate fusional potential has been suggested as a method of improving the results of initial surgery and minimising the rate of reoperation. A prospective, randomised multicentre clinical trial was performed (Prism adaptation study research group, *Arch Ophthalmol*, 108, 1248-56, 1990).

"The results indicated that prism adaptation better defines the target angle of surgery and results in a higher rate of satisfactory alignment without an increased risk of over correction. It is particularly useful for those patients who build up larger angles and then undergo surgery for the adapted angle" (Tony Murray, 1993)[17].

To finally sum up, in cases of concomitant squint, the management could be summarised in Chart 10.1.

Chart 10.1

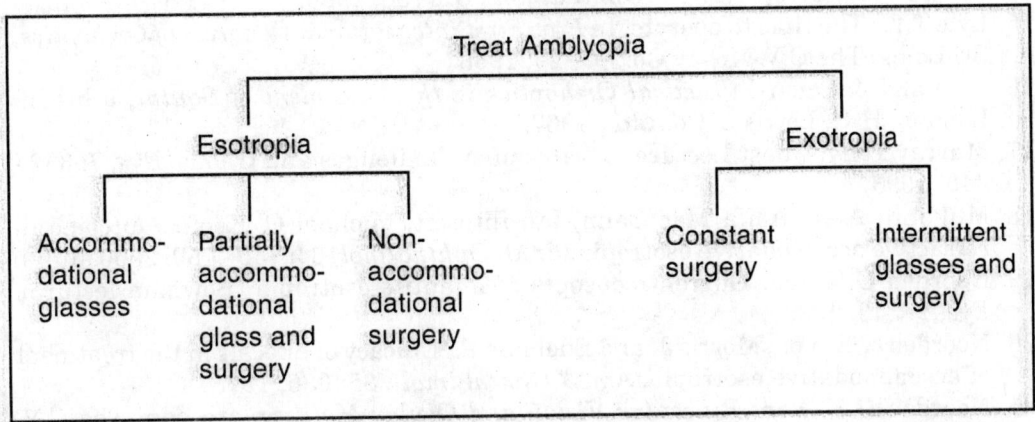

REFERENCES

1. Archer S.M Helveston E.M. et al: Stereopsis in normal infants and infants with congenital esotropia. *Am. J. Ophthalmol*, 101:591,1986.
2. Baker J.D and Parks M.M: Early onset accommodative esotropia. *Am J. Ophthalmol.*, 90:11,1980.
3. Chavasse F.B.: *Worth's Squint or the Binocular Reflexes and the Treatment of Strabismus,* 7th edn. London, Bailliere Tindall and Cox, 1939, p. 519.
4. Costenbader F.D, Ing M., Bair R.V and Parks M.M.: Symposium Infantile esotropia. *Am. Orthopt.*, 18:5, 1968.
5. Crone R.A : From orthophoria to microtropia. *Brit. Orthopt. J.*, 26:45,1969.
6. Duke-Elder S.W. *Text Book of Ophthalmology*, Vol. IV, London, Henry Kimpton, 1949.
7. Gittoes-Davies R.: An examination of the etiology and treatment of small convergent deviation associated with a low degree of hypermetropia. *Br. Orthopt. J.*, 8:71, 1951.
8. Helveston E.M., Ellis F. D., Schott J. Mitchelson J., Weber J. C., Traube S. and Miller K.: Surgical treatment of congenital esotropia. *Am.J. Ophthalmol.*, 96:218, 1983.
9. Helveston E.M. and Noorden G.K. Von: Microtropia: A newly defined entity. *Arch. Ophthalmol.*, 78:272, 1967.
10. Hiles D. A. Watson A. Biglam A. W.: Characteristics of infantile esotropia following early bimedial rectus recession. *Arch Ophthamol*, 98: 697 - 703, 1988.
11. Ingram R.M, Walker C, Wilson J.M, Arnold P. E. Lucas J. and Dally S.: A first attempt to prevent amblyopia and squint by spectacle correction of abnormal refraction from age 1 year *Brit. J. Ophthalmol.*, 69: 851,1983.

12. Keenan J M. Willshaw H E: The outcome of strabismus surgery in childhood esotropia. Eye, 7, 341 - 345, 1993.

13. Jampolsky A: Differential diagnosis and management of small degree esotropia and convergent fixation-disparity. *Am. J. Ophthalmol.*, 41: 825,1956..

14. Lang J.: Microtropia. *Arch. Ophthalmol.*, 81: 758, 1969.

15. Lyle T.K.: The time to operate. In *Proc First International Congress of Orthoptics*, St. Louis, The C.V Mosby Co., p. 129, 1968.

16. Lyle and Jacksons' *Practical Orthoptics in the Treatment of Squint*, 5th edn. London, H.K. Lewis & Co. Ltd., 1967.

17. Murray Tony: Guest Lecture - strabismus: Challenges and trends. *Eye*, 7: 332 - 340, 1993.

18. Mulvihill Alan, Aoifa Mac Cann, Ian fliteroft, Michael O' Keefe: Outcome in refractive accomodative esotropia. *Br. J. Ophthalmol*, 84: 746 - 759, 2000 (July).

19. Noorden G.K Von: Current concepts of infantile esotropia (Bowman lecture). *Eye*, 2: 343, 1988.

20. Noorden G.K. Von, Morris J. and Edelman P.: Efficacy of bifocals in the treatment of accommodative esotropia. *Am. J.Ophthalmol.*, 85: 830, 1978.

21. Noorden G.K. Von: *Binocular Vision and Ocular Motility*, 4th edn. The C.V. Mosby Company, St. Louis, 1990.

22. Parks M.M.: Abnormal accommodative convergence in squint. Arch. Ophthalmol., 59: 364, 1958.

23. Rohatgi J.N., Prasad C.M., Prasad B.K. and Kumar A.: Concomitant alternating squint. *Indian J. Ophthalmol.*, 27 iv:141,1979.

24. Scott A.B.: Botulinum toxin injection into extra-ocular muscle, as an alternative to strabismus surgery. *Ophthalmology*, 87: 1044,1980.

25. Setayesh A.R., Khodadoust A.A. and Daryani S.M.: Microtropia. *Arch. Ophthalmol.*, 96:1842, 1978.

26. Taylor D.M.: Congenital strabismus, the common sense approach. *Arch. Ophthalmol.*, 77: 1967.

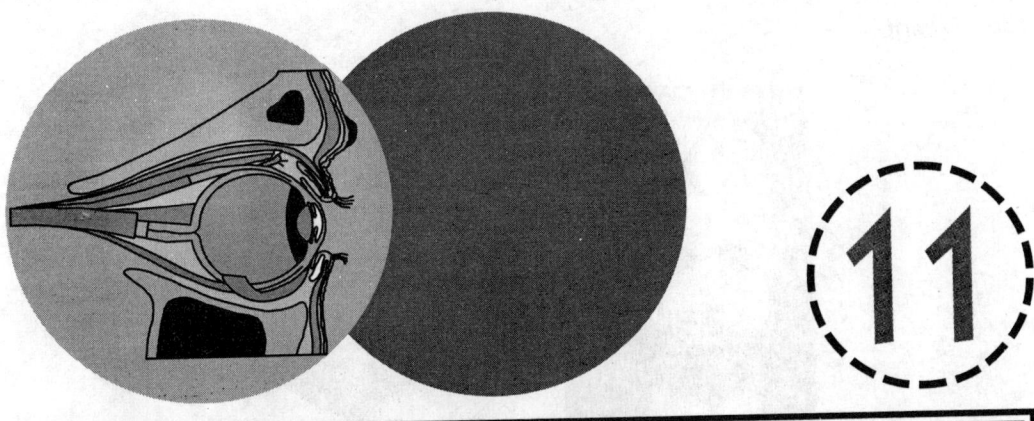

Concomitant–Divergent Strabismus
Exotropia

Divergent squints are less common than the convergent ones, a rough ratio of 1 to 4. They tend to develop slowly and the angle of deviation increases gradually as age advances. They are more common in a latent or intermittent form than are esodeviation. The deviation appears first as an intermittent squint, the degree of deviation being variable and averaging some 20° in ordinary circumstances (Fig. 11.1).

A patient may exihibit a manifest exotropia during one examination and at the next sitting an exophoria or intermittent exotropia may be seen. To some extent, these deviations are frequently controllable. The patient may straighten his visual axis and exercise fusion by an effort of will and only to allow the eye to wander out when his attention lapses. The deviation may appear to increase on upward regard and to decrease on looking down due to mechanical conditions favouring divergence on elevation of the eyes and convergence on depression.

Alternation is more often found than amongst convergent squints, more so, in the cases where intermittency is the primary deviation pattern. And suppression is the usual expedient adopted to achieve visual comfort. This eliminates diplopia.

The prognosis for recovery of binocular function is better in those who experience a long phase of intermittency than in those with a manifest deviation since early childhood, and in those where the deviation is constant.

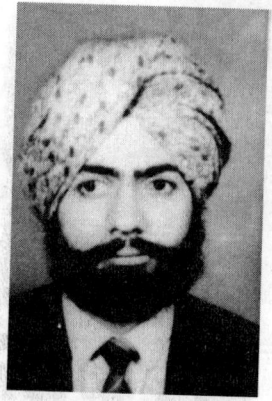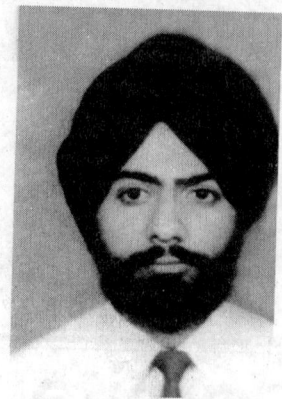

Fig. 11.1: *Right divergent squint in a young man before and after operation.*

A useful clinical classification of concomitant exotropia is: (a) Primary divergent squint, (b) secondary divergent squints, and (c) consecutive divergent squint. Paralytic divergent squint resulting from paresis/paralysis of the medial rectus muscle is outside the scope of this discussion.

PRIMARY DIVERGENT SQUINT

Where the deviation is constant or intermittent can be subdivided into (Duane's[7] classification, Noorden[16]) the following patterns (Figs 11.2 A and B).

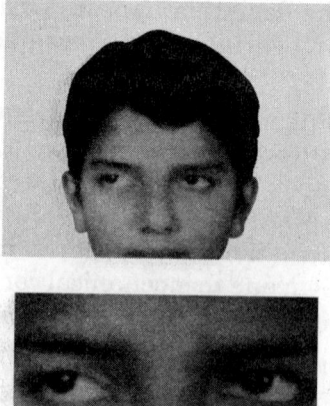

Fig. 11.2 A: *A case of alternating divergent squint in a school-going boy of 12 years for operation. Right eye fixing and left eye diverging.*

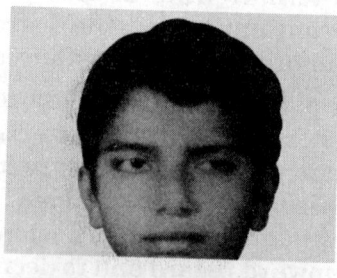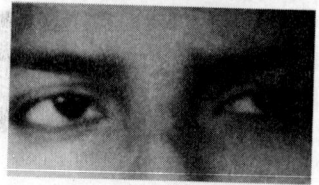

Fig. 11.2 B: *Same case as in Fig. 11.2. Left eye fixing and right eye diverging.*

i. *Divergent excess pattern:* The divergence or exodeviation is more apparent when looking at a distant object (and not fixing attention on anything particular) and is at least 15 Δ larger than at near-fixation (viewing a near object) as seen in Fig. 11.3.

ii. *Convergence weakness pattern:* The divergence occurs essentially when the patient is looking at a near object and the near deviation is at least 15 Δ greater than the distance-deviation.

iii. *Basic-mixed deviation:* The distance deviation is more or less equal to near deviation. The deviation may occur in any circumstance without relation to the proximity or remoteness of the objects of regard (Figs 11.2 A & B).

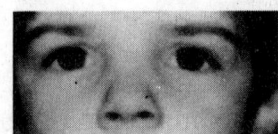 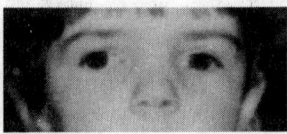

Fig. 11.3: *Exotropia of the excess pattern divergence.*

Etiology

Normally the visual axes are maintained in parallelism owing to the constant expenditure of tonic-convergence to overcome the anatomically determined exophoria. The position of the eyes is one of divergence and as growth occurs, particularly about puberty, the divergence of the orbital axes tends to accentuate with a decrease of tonic-convergence. As age increases, fusion-impulse becomes weak or its amplitude decreases and thus, manifest divergence tends to appear. At times, the fusion-faculty is weak, not fully developed so that the fusional coordination of the eyes is poor and readily disrupted. And as such the tendency to develop a divergent position (squint) gradually increases with age in these cases (Duke Elder[8]).

In the usual type of acquired myopia (of about 5–6 dioptres) the near point of clear vision approaches the eye. Accommodation is required to a decreasing extent and so the synergic element of convergence is not stimulated proportionately. An external deviation or exodeviation is evident in most of these myopes. In later life when the near-point of distinct vision recedes and convergence is still less required, the tendency to divergence increases and may become manifest.

Such a divergent-squint is not very marked (15° to 20°) and is variable, sometimes disappearing in distant vision and increasing with fatigue or illness. As the potentiality of fusion is frequently retained, the deviation tends to be alternating rather than uniocular. Good vision is thus being retained in each eye.

In uncorrected astigmatism and in extreme hypermetropia when accommodation fails to provide a clear vision, it is given up. As a result or sequence the convergence suffers from disuse. It is not required and an alternating manifest divergence tends to result.

Symptomatology

Patients with exophoria commonly complain of eyestrain and blurring of vision. They experience difficulty with prolonged periods of reading, these being headache and occasional diplopia. Those with constant exotropia are less symptomatic. The intermittent ones have the same complaints of asthenopia. The most common complaint is that of deviation itself which causes social embarrasment.

Examination and Investigation

The onset of squint is usually early in life. A careful history has to be taken to elicit whether the exodeviation began as intermittent or has been constant from the very beginning. This determines the line of management.

Visual acuity and refractive error-with unilateral and constant deviation, the visual acuity in the squinting eye may be defective. It is normal and more or less equal in cases with alternating exotropia-intermittent or constant.

Recent studies[2,10] have shown that the etiology of the divergent concomitant squint is unrelated to the underlying refractive error. And that the distribution of refractive error in these cases is more or less similar to that in the corresponding age non-squinting population. Some of the cases are of acquired myopia (*as explained above*) or of myopic astigmatism.

A well-developed suppression mechanism in the non-fixing squinting eye eliminates diplopia and is a common finding in alternating cases. In patients with the divergence excess type of exodeviation, a latent strabismus at near-fixation often coexists with a manifest strabismus at distance-fixation. Thus in these cases normal binocular vision is constantly being reinforced and sensory adaptations are not infrequent. Impaired binocular visual acuity may be due to the overexercise of convergence and consequently of accommodation in order to achieve control of the deviation.

Cover-test (Lyle[15]) It should be elicited both for near (1/3 metre), distance (6 metre) and also for distance beyond 6 metres. Depending on the type of divergent squint, it may give the following information.

i. At near-distance of 1/3 metre the cover-test may show manifest divergence or latent divergence with a varying rate of recovery to binocular single vision or at times without any spontaneous recovery.

ii. At 6 metre distance the cover-test may show the same findings as at 1/3rd metre. The patient reads the 6/9 line on Snellen chart and thereby, keeps his accommodation relaxed and with it the convergence.

iii. At beyond 6 metre distance the deviation may be manifest or latent. A large angle of deviation may be detected and the fusional state of the patient may be revealed under a more natural visual condition.

i. In cases of divergence-excess type of intermittent divergent squint, which is more common the divergence is pronounced for distance fixation at 6 metres or beyond. At the near distance of 1/3rd meter, it may show some divergence or no divergence (depending on the degree of divergence) Divergence is less marked for near than for distance-fixation on account of the accommodation and associated convergence which are brought into play when looking at a near object. If, however, full dissociation is allowed to occur and careful measurement is then made which enables accommodation to be relaxed, the full amount of deviation for the near is revealed and the angle of deviation for near and distance fixation may be found to be approximately equal.

Unilaterally occluding one eye for one hour (Burian[2] prefers it for 30 to 45 minutes) and then measuring the deviation both for distance and near-fixation is sufficient to show increase in the near deviation. Occlusion removes the binocular fusion stimulation.

This is simulated divergence excess pattern of exodeviation when the static deviation at near-fixation is obscured by dynamic factors such as persistent convergence innervation. Kushner (1999)[4] mentions "patients with exotropia often have a slow-to-dissipate fusional mechanism at near which masks the true near deviation. Consequently, determination of the accommodation-convergence accommodation (Ac/A) ratio in patients with exotropia must be based on near measurement obtained after prolonged monocular occlusion (typically 1 hour).

When determined in this manner, the presence of a high Ac/A ratio before surgery in an exotropic patient has been reported to be predictive of an esophoria at near distance after surgery. And such a patient may need a bifocal after surgery for control of the near esotropia.

Proper identification can thus, permit forewarning of the patient who is at risk for needing a bifocal after surgery. In also indicates patients who are good candidates for overcorrecting with minus lens therapy.

Further when Ac/A ratio seems high with heterophoria method (after 1 hour of mono-ocular occlusion), the possible effect of proximal convergence must be ruled out by a gradient method determination.

ii. In cases of long standing divergent squint- a super-added convergence deficiency may cause the angle of deviation to be greater for near than for distance (convergence deficiency type).

iii. In basic type cover-test shows the divergence both at near and distance fixation to be more or less the same.

The cover-test should be carried out in various cardinal directions of gaze, specially on looking directly upwards and downwards. This may elicit the presence of A and V syndrome.

State of Binocular Single Vision

i. In patients with the Divergence-excess type of exotropia, a latent strabismus at near-fixation often coexists with a manifest divergence at distance-fixation. In such a situation, binocular single vision is constantly being reinforced at least for near-distance. As such, amblyopia with eccentric-fixation is rare. Similarly abnormal retinal correspondence (ARC) does not occur in these cases.

Amblyopia and ARC are likely findings in cases with constant unilateral exotropia.

ii. In patients with intermittent exotropia normal and abnormal correspondence may coexist.

iii. In alternating type of exotropia, with more or less normal visual acuity in each eye, there is suppression of the non-fixing eye.

Treatment

Optical

Refraction has to be assessed under full cycloplegia and the correct glasses prescribed. Full correction is advisable in myopic patients to maintain as also stimulate accommodational convergence. This helps to control and or to mask the exodeviation.

Astigmatism and anisometropia have to be corrected to produce sharp retinal images, which in turn would increase the stimulus to fuse.

Since correction of any hypermetropic refractive-error will decrease the demand on accommodation-convergence and this may increase the exodeviation, each patient should be evaluated on an individual basis. Children with hypermetropia of less than + 2.00 dioptre need no correction.

Surgical Treatment

Three factors have to be taken into account before deciding for surgery in exotropia, viz. (1) angle size of deviation, (2) the age of the patient, and (3) the state of fusional control (Noorden[16], Pratt-Johnson[18]).

  a. In young children with constant exotropia right from birth or shortly after birth and with no history of intermittency and when the deviation is more than 15° (25 Δ) surgery should be undertaken to correct the deviation as soon as possible after reliable measurements of the deviation are obtainable. This could be possible between 1 and 2 years of age, otherwise chances for development of amblyopia and loss of stereopsis are there.

b. In adults again with a large angle of deviation and constant deviation, surgery is indicated at the earliest. The prognosis for return of normal binocular function is poor in those cases where the deviation has been present from early childhood. The operative straightening of the eyes is a cosmetic cure. But at times, it has been the experience that even in some cases of late surgery, unexpected return of binocular single vision with stereopsis has occurred.

c. Where the deviation is intermittent or has become constant after a long period of intermittency, surgery may be delayed and efforts directed to improve the binocular function. Efforts have to be made to eliminate amblyopia or eradicate suppression by means of alternate occlusion and by orthoptic exercises (with synoptophore) and reinforcing fusion with minus lenses.

Even in those cases, where regular examination shows an increase in the size of basic-deviation or development of suppression (as evidenced by absence of diplopia) during the manifest phase of strabismus, surgery should be considered.

(2) The desirable age at which surgery should be done in case of intermittent exotropia is a matter of opinion Jampolsky (1962)[13] prefers to delay surgery in infants to avoid overcorrection. Knapp[14] (1958, 1971) on the other hand is an advocate for early surgery.

Surgical Results

Getting back to the binocular function or conversion from a manifest divergence to latent exophoria, depends on the binocular state before surgery and this is unpredictable and variable. Then in some cases, with large angles of deviation, there is the problem of undercorrection which needs additional surgery. Use of base-in membrane prisms of a dioptric value greater than the residual deviation has been advocated to provoke convergence and thereby, lessen the angle of deviation.

The criteria for satisfactory treatment in these cases of primary divergent squint are (Lyle[15]).

   i. The patient is symptom-free.
  ii. There is no manifest deviation. A small degree of latent deviation may be demonstrable on cover test but there is rapid recovery.
 iii. Normal binocular function should be demonstrable.
  iv. Binocular visual acuity for near and distance fixation with glass (if any) should be as good as the visual acuity of the less efficient eye.

SECONDARY DIVERGENT SQUINT

When the development of binocular single is obstructed by factors which may be congenital or acquired, secondary divergent concomitant squint may result.

Such obstacles may be sensory or motor in nature. An example of such a sensory obstacle is seen in cases of corneal leucoma, traumatic unilateral cataract, optic atropy, etc. when the vision in the affected eye is very much reduced. The same factors in a child below the age of 5 years may produce an esodeviation but developing in adolescence or in adult, they produce exodeviation.

In adults, there is another typical example of unilateral aphakia which if not taken care of, causes divergence in that eye.

The onset of presbyopia sometimes accelerates the rate of divergence because with the decrease in the power of accommodation there may be a corresponding weakness of convergence.

The aim of treatment in these cases is to improve the ocular appearance which is possible only with surgery aiming at a slight overcorrection. Successful surgery may improve distance stereoacuity. Better distance stereoacuity and central fusion are frequently associated with better surgical success (Cem Yildirim, 1999) [6].

Motor Obstacle

Divergence is more often associated with a primary paresis of the superior or inferior rectus muscle.

In oxycephaly because of less space in orbit, the visual axes show a divergent strabismus.

CONSECUTIVE DIVERGENT SQUINT

This may result from (i) overliberal surgical correction of a convergent squint specially if binocular function is defective or absent, or (ii) it may occur spontaneously in certain cases of convergent squint specially if the deviating eye is amblyopic from high hypermetropic refractive error. The hypermetropia is present only in the deviating eye.

These cases are problems for cosmetic surgery of the deviation.

REFERENCES

1. Burian H.M. Intermittent (facultative) divergent strabismus, its influence on visual acuity and binocular visual act. *Am.J.Ophthalmol.*, 28: 525, 1945.
2. Burian H.M.: Exodeviations: their classification, diagnosis and treatment. *Am.J.Ophthalmol.*, 62:1161, 1966.
3. Burian H.M. and Spivey B.E.: The Surgical management of exodeviations. *Am.J.Ophthalmol.*, 59: 603, 1965.
4. Burton J. Kushner M D: Diagnosis and treatment of exotropia with a high accommodation-convergence-accommodation ratio. *Arch Ophthalmol.*, 117: 221-224 1999.

5. Chavasse F.E.: *Worth's Squint or the Binocular Reflexes and the Treatment of Strabismus.* London, Bailliere Tindall and Cox, 1939.
6. Cem Yildirim et al: Assessment of central and peripheral fusion and near and distance stereoacuity in intermittent exotropic patients before and after strabismus surgery. *Am. J. Ophthalmol,* 128: 222 - 230 1999.
7. Duane A: A new classification of the motor anomalies of the eyes based upon physiological principles, together with their symptoms, diagnosis and treatment. *Ann.Ophthalmol.Otolaryngol.,* 5:969/1896:6:84 and 247,1897.
8. Duke-Elder S.: *Textbook of Ophthalmology,* Vol.4. London, Henry Kimpton, 1949.
9. Eustace P., Wesson M.E. and Druby D.J.: The effect of illumination on intermittent divergent squint of the divergence excess type. *Trans Ophthalmol,* UK, 93: 559: 1973.
10. Hall I.B.: Primary divergent strabismus- analysis of etiological factors. *Br.Orthoph.J.,* 18:106,1961.
11. Hardesty H H. Boynton J.R. and Keenan J.P.: Treatment of intermittent exotropia. *Arch Ophthalmol.,* 96: 268, 1978.
12. Hiles B. A., Davies G.T and Costenbader F.D. Long-term observations on unoperated intermittent exotropia. *Arch. Ophthalmol.,* 80: 436, 1968.
13. Jampolsky, A: Surgical management of exotropia. *Am. J. Ophthalmol.,* 46: 646, 1958.
14. Knapp P.: Management of exotropia: In symposium on strabismus. *Trans. New Orleans Academy of Ophthalmology,* St. Louis, C.V. Mosby Co., 1971.
15. Lyle and Jackson's *Practical Orthoptics in the Treatment of Squint,* 5th edn. London, H.K. Lewis and Co. Ltd., 1967.
16. Noorden G.K. Von: *Binocular Vision and Ocular Motility,* 4th edn. St. Louis C.V. Mosby Company, 1990.
17. Parks, M.M: Comitant exodeviation in children. In *Strabismus Symposium of the New Orleans Academy of Ophthalmology.* St. Louis, The C. V. Mosby Co., 1962.
18. Pratt-Johnson J. A., Barlow J.M. and Tilson G: Early surgery for intermittent exotropia. *Am. J. Ophthalmol.,* 84:869, 1977.
19. Rohatgi J.N., Bimal Chandra: Intermittent Exotropia, *Proc. 44th All India Ophthalmological Society,* Kanpur, 1986, page 293-296.
20. Scholssman A. and Boruchoff S.A. Correlation between physiologic and clinical aspects of exotropia. *Am. J. Ophthalmol.,* 40: 53, 1955.
21. Scott W.E. and Mash A.J. The postoperative results and stability of exodeviations. *Arch Ophthalmol.,* 99:1814, 1981.
22. Wang F.M. and Chryssanthou G. Ocular eye closure in intermittent exotropia. *Arch Ophthalmol.,* 106: 941, 1988.

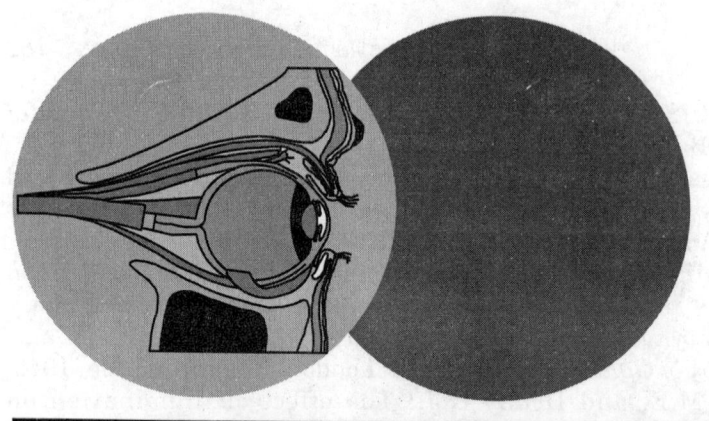

A and V Syndrome

A simple observation that a horizontal deviation may increase or decrease with the eyes in upward and downward gaze was not noticed carefully or given any clinical significance in management till 1948, when Uretts-Zavatia (quoted in Noorden[10]) published his first paper.

In his paper, the author emphasised the importance of measuring the angle of deviation (in cases of strabismus) in the straight upward and downward positions of gaze in addition to the usual measurement in the primary straight ahead position of seeing.

Three years later, Urist[13] in 1951, in his paper published in *Archives of Ophthalmology*, drew attention to cases of horizontal concomitant squint with secondary vertical deviations. Since then discussions started in American literature, and in 1957 Albert D[1] suggested the excellent descriptive term of A-pattern and V-pattern. These deviations have also been described as A and V phenomena or A and V syndrome. They indicate that there is a considerable difference in the angle of the horizontal deviation on looking upwards (supraversion) as compared with looking downwards (infraversion).

Classification

A-pattern indicates a considerable increase in the angle of convergence (or decrease in the angle of divergence) with upwards gaze and *V-pattern* indicate those cases showing a considerable increase in the angle of convergence (or decrease in the angle of divergence) on downward gaze. A working classification of these patterns is as follows (Fig. 12.1).

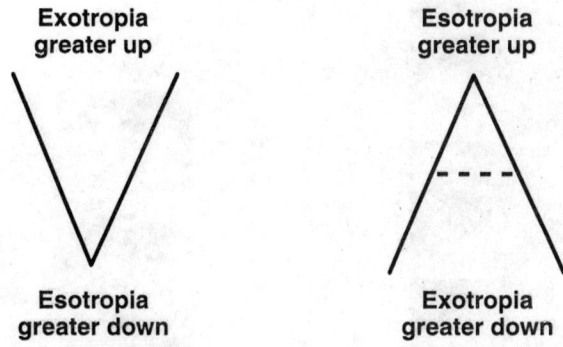

Exotropia
greater up

Esotropia
greater up

Esotropia
greater down

Exotropia
greater down

Fig 12.1: *Line representation of A and V syndrome/pattern.*

I. *A-pattern*

a. *A-Esotropia (esophoria)* In A esotropia/esophoria (Fig. 12.2). The convergent deviation increases in direct upward gaze and decreases in downward gaze.

b. *A-Exotropia (exophoria)* Here the divergent deviation increases in downward gaze than when looking directly upwards (Fig. 12.3).

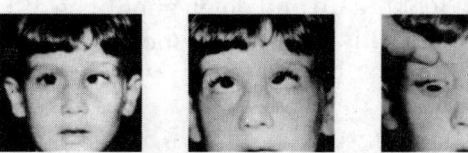

Fig 12.2: *A case of A pattern esotropia. Left hand figure left eye esotropia-case in primary position. Middle figure shows increased esotropia in upward gaze while right hand figure normal alignment in downward gaze.*

II. *V-pattern*

a. *V-Esotropia/esophoria,* The convergent deviation is greater when looking directly downwards than when looking directly upwards (Fig. 12.4).

b. *V-Exotropia/exophoria,* The divergent deviation is considerably greater on looking directly upwards than when looking directly downwards (Fig. 12.5).

Besides these symptoms, there are patients who may show no deviation or only a small deviation in the primary straight ahead position, but may show exotropia both in the upward and downwards gaze (X-pattern).

Again exotropia may be present only in the upward gaze (Y-pattern) or in the downward gaze (Lambda pattern). They are considered as modifications of the classical A and V-pattern (Noorden[10]).

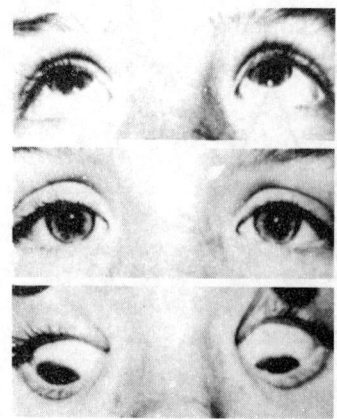

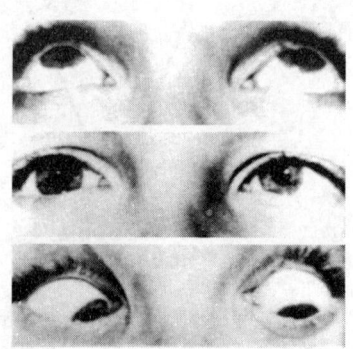

Fig 12.3: *In upward gaze orthophoria. In primary position no deviation. In downward gaze marked exotropia.*

Fig 12.4: *In upward gaze slight exotropia. Central figure Primary gaze esotropia, In downward gaze increased esotropia.*

A certain degree of V-deviations are considered physiological for when we look upwards (supraversion); there is a slight relative divergence and when we look downwards (infraversion) there is a slight relative convergence. Therefore it has been suggested that to be labelled as cases of V-phenomena, the difference in the angle of deviation on looking up and down should be at least 15 Δ Whereas and in cases of A-phenomena this difference should be at least 10 Δ (prism dioptre).

Etiology

The exact pathophysiology of cases of AV syndrome is conjectural. Three groups of etiological factors are described on

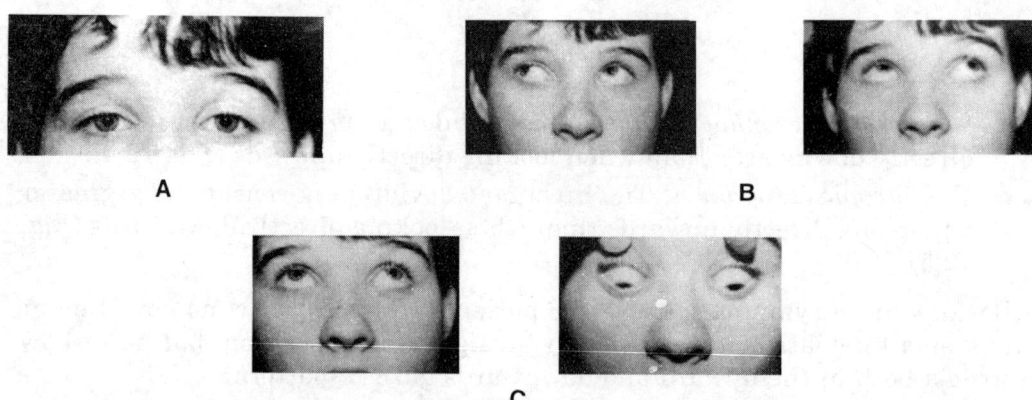

Fig 12.5: *A case of V exotropia. **A** Eyes in primary position with no deviation. **B** Exotropia in up right gaze and up left gaze. **C** Left upward gaze and right downward gaze.*

1. The horizontal school of Urist[13, 15] (1951-1958),
2. vertical school of Brown[3] (1963), and
3. oblique school.

Brown[3] was of the opinion that A and V patterns may be caused by primary anomalies in the functioning of vertical rectus muscles. But since overaction and under action of the oblique muscles are frequently associated with A and V syndrome, it soon came to be realised that the vertical and oblique muscles jointly are responsible for these changes in the angle of deviation when looking upwards and downwards. Hence, it is suggested that the etiological factors could be discussed into two groups of (1) horizontal school, and (2) vertical school combining the vertical and oblique schools in one as follows.

The Horizontal School of Urist [13, 15] (1951- 58)

Urist thought that A and V patterns/syndromes are the results of abnormal action of the horizontal recti muscles. According to him, overaction of the lateral rectus muscle causes an increased relative divergence when looking upwards (upwards gaze). And an overaction of the medial rectus muscle causes increased relative convergence in downward gaze.

Similarly, an underaction of the lateral rectus muscle may cause an increased relative convergence in upward gaze and an underaction of the medial rectus muscle may cause an increased relative divergence in downward gaze. And thus, the V-pattern esophoria/esotropia) is the result of an overacting medial rectus muscle and the V- pattern exophoria (exotropia) is the result of an overacting lateral rectus muscle. On the other hand, an underacting lateral rectus muscle causes A esophoria (esotropia) and an underacting medial rectus muscle causes A exophoria (exotropia)

The Vertical School of Brown

According to this, these A and V pattern cases result from a symmetrical underaction of the vertically acting muscles (Lyle[8]).

In V-phenomenon, it seems likely that the basic defect is weakness of superior oblique muscle with a consequent overaction of the inferior rectus muscle in the opposite eye. This takes the eye downward. As superior oblique muscles is weak, its tertiary action of abduction is decreased, the eye remains relatively more convergent and adducted facilitating the depression of the globe by an overacting inferior rectus muscle.

The ipsilateral inferior oblique overacts causing an abduction of the globe on elevation in a relatively less convergent or more divergent position in upward gaze. (inferior oblique secondary action is elevation and tertiary action abduction). And thus, one gets a V-phenomenon with esophoria/ esotropia.

The A pattern similarly can be explained on the basis of a weak inferior oblique muscle with consequent overaction of the superior rectus muscle in the other eye (Contra lateral synergist muscle). A weak inferior oblique favours adduction (or less abduction, the tertiary action of inferior oblique) and a overacting superior rectus favours abduction and elevation. So the eye tends to converge in adduction, A esotropia/esophoria. At the same time, an overacting superior oblique in the same eye (ipsilateral anatagonist muscle) causes abduction of the eye in depression. This produces A extropia/exophoria.

Thus, a combination of vertical and oblique muscles overaction and underaction can explain the A and V pattern. To explain these on the basis of only the vertical recti muscles or only on the basis of the oblique muscles, under- and overaction is rather puzzling or mind boggling and a pure academic exercise.

Oplique School

That these patterns are the result of combined abnormalities of action of the horizontal and vertically acting muscles.

It seems likely that when these patterns are present to a slight degree, the cause is an abnormal action of the horizontal recti and it is also possible that an abnormality of both the vertical and horizontal muscles may be operative in certain cases. It has been pointed out that the A pattern tends to occur in people with a mongoloid type of face with high cheek bones and palpebral fissure with upward slope.

The shape of the orbit in this type of anomaly of the skull may predispose to a relative underaction of the inferior oblique with overaction of the superior oblique thus, resulting in relative divergence on looking downwards.

On the other hand the V pattern may occur in people with anti-mongoloid face, flat cheek bones and palpebral fissure with downward slope in which the shape of the orbit may predispose to a relative underaction of the superior oblique with overaction of the inferior oblique, thus, resulting in relative divergence on looking upwards.

Anomalies of Muscle Insertion

Weiss (1966) as quoted by Noorden[10] attributed the A and V patterns to the action of the abnormally inserted superior and inferior rectus muscles and the upshoot and downshoot in adduction to the action of the abnormally inserted medial rectus muscle.

The clinician is thus, in lurch about the pathogenesis of the A and V patterns and, therefore, confused about the appropriate surgical decision when planning operation in these cases. Should primary surgical procedure be performed on oblique muscles or should horizontal muscles be operated on before the oblique muscle? His own clinical judgement is the best arbiter in such a situation.

Clinical Features and Diagnosis

An increase of deviation in downward gaze (with A exotropia and V esotropia) may cause discomfort during reading or the near work. On the other hand an increase of deviation in the upward gaze (V exotropia) may not be evident to the patient since little or no interference with binocular single vision would occur in the functionally more important primary or downward position of viewing.

A case of convergent squint showing a V pattern may be mistaken as a case of accommodative convergence excess type of deviation and vice versa for in both of these conditions in distance fixation (looking slightly upward) there may be binocular-single vision whereas, in near fixation (in the reading position) looking slightly downward there may be a manifest convergent squint.

It is also possible that the V-pattern in divergent strabismus (V-exotropia) may be confused with divergence excess type of exotropia in which a wider divergence of the visual axes is prone to occur in upward gaze.

Hence, the deviation should be measured in three sets viz. (1) in primary position looking straight ahead, (ii) looking upwards 25° of upward gaze, and (iii) looking down wards 25° of downward gaze.

The ocular movements have to be carefully analysed in all the cardinal positions to detect any paresis of a horizontal or vertical ocular muscle. For this an examination on Hess screen may also be utilised.

In a V pattern is which the difference in deviation between upward and downward gaze is 15Δ (prism-dioptre) or more should be considered a significant vertical incommitancy.

On the other hand an A pattern (which is never found as a normal variant) a limit of 10 Δ (prism-dioptre) has been set beyond which an A pattern is thought to be significant. Thus an A exotropia with only 15 Δ deviation in downward gaze and 5 Δ in primary position may interfere with normal binocular vision and needs treatment.

Chin elevation and depression with a horizontal deviation should be carefully looked for. Thus, one with A esotropia and V exotropia may hold his chin in an elevated position and conversely a child with V esotropia and A exotropia may show chin depression.

Treatment

It is indicated when binocular vision is disturbed. This is more common in cases of A exotropia and V esotropia, and the treatment is surgery.

It may not be indicated for the simple purpose of decreasing a cosmetically acceptable deviation in upward gaze in a patient who is asymptomatic with his eyes in the primary straight ahead position and in the downward gaze.

Corrective unilateral or bilateral surgical procedures for horizontal squints combined with, preceded by, or followed by weakening and strengthening procedures on the oblique muscles have proved effective in most patients with A and V syndrome to correct the vertical incomitance.

Transposition of Horizontal and Vertical Recti Muscles

The effect of surgery on horizontal recti can be enhanced or decreased in upward and downward gaze by vertical transposition of the insertion of the horizontal recti muscles. This technique was described by Knapp[7] in (1969).

Thus, when the insertion of the medial rectus is lowered, its horizontal action decreases in downward gaze. As for the lateral rectus, when its insertion is raised, the horizontal action is decreased in elevation (see chapter 8).

In practice, therefore, based on theoretical considerations one can proceed as follows.

In cases of esotropia — convergent position of the eye.

a. *V esotropia* (Clinically more commonly met with) a recession of the medial rectus along with lowering its insertion. This may be combined with resection of lateral rectus and lowering its insertion.

b. *A esotropia* a recession of medial rectus alongwith raising its insertion. This may be combined with resection of lateral rectus and lowering its insertion.

In cases of exotropia — divergent position of the eye

a. *V exotropia* (again clinically more common) a recession of lateral rectus alongwith raising its insertion, along with medial rectus resection and raising its insertion.

b. *A exotropia* is less frequent clinically. The deviation can be corrected by lateral rectus recession. This may be combined with medial rectus resection and raising its insertion.

Thus it can be said as follows (Noorden[10]).

a. When the overaction of a muscle is to be neutralised, besides recession, move the insertion in the direction in which weakening or neutralisation is required (decreased action), and

b. When the underaction has to be strengthened, besides resection move the insertion in the direction opposite in which strengthening is required (increase in action or more effectivity).

c. When performing resection/recession procedure on a patient who also has a small to moderate vertical deviation, both horizontal muscles may be shifted vertically. This approach can treat the vertical component or deviation without altering the effects of the procedure for the eso- or exo-deviation. The muscles are moved upwards, if the eye is hypodeviated and downwards if the eye is hyperdeviated. The amount of movement upwards and downwards shall not exceed one half of muscle width.

But since in these cases of A and V syndrome, the oblique muscles along with the vertical recti also play an important role, each case has to be analysed to ascertain the action of horizontal, vertical and oblique muscles and surgery is planned accordingly.

Thus, in cases with inferior oblique overaction, along with horizontal recti as in cases of V-esotropia and V-exotropia, one could proceed as follows.

I. (a) In cases of V-esotropia and overacting inferior oblique, an inferior oblique weakening procedure will diminish the V pattern in upward gaze. Combined to this, a weakening procedure on the medical rectus may be all that is necessary to bring the eye to normal parallelism- (MR recession and downward displacement of the insertion.

(b) On the other hand in cases of V exotropia: A weakening procedure on inferior oblique muscle decreases the deviation in upward gaze and this may be sufficient to create a satisfactory functional result. If, however, there is a left over significant amount of exodeviation in primary and downward positions of gaze, surgery on horizontal muscle becomes a necessity, lateral rectus recession and, if necessary, also an upward displacement of the lateral rectus insertion.

II. In cases of (a) A esotropia with superior oblique overaction a weakening procedure on superior oblique may be necessary and thereafter, to prevent exotropia in downward gaze or in primary position, horizontal muscle surgery has to be done. Resection of the lateral rectus and lowering of its insertion.

(b) In cases of A exotropia — again with superior oblique overaction, bilateral weakening procedure on superior oblique along with surgery on horizontal muscle may be performed, resection of MR and upward displacement of its insertion.

And hence to achieve success in these cases one has to carefully evaluate and analyse the degree of deviation in the primary-straight ahead position and on looking upwards and downwards before deciding whether to tackle the horizontal muscle only or to have a two stage surgery on the horizontal muscles and involving the vertical/muscle also, as the case may warrant.

Stanworth[12] (1968), while writing about the A and V syndrome, (in the *British Journal of Orthoptic* Vol.26, page 12-28,1969) has very lucidly described the possible surgical treatment in these patterns (Table 12.1).

But to get unanimity amongst surgeons, who combine the vertical/oblique muscle surgery along with horizontal muscles is not forthcoming. Thus, Shin GS et al[18] of Jules Sten Eye Institute, Los Angeles, suggested posterior superior oblique tenectomy at the scleral insertion for collapse of A pattern, whereas Forster[19] suggested unilateral tucking and advancement of inferior oblique muscle for the treatment of A pattern.

Table 12.1

1. A-Esotropia	Resection or tucking IO Tenotomy SO .	Recession of IO	Resection lateral rectus	Move LR insertion downwards	Antero position of SO	Temporal Transplant of SO
2. A-Exotropia	Resection of IR Tenotomy SO		Resection of MR	Move MR insertion upwards		Medial transplant IR
3. V-Esotropia	Resection of IO or myectomy tucking of SO	Antero position of IO muscle	Recession MR.	Medial Rectus insertion down.	Antero position of IO	Temporal TransPlant IR
4. V-Exotropia	Recession or myectomy IO Resection of SR		Recession LR	Move LR insertion upwards		Medial transplant of SR

NOTE: NB MR Medial rectus muscle   SO Superior oblique muscle
LR Lateral rectus muscle   IO Inferior oblique muscle.

REFERENCES

1. Albert D.G. Personal Communication in Parks MM Annual review strabismus, *Arch Ophthalmol*, 58:152,1957
2. Billet E. and Freedman M.: Surgery of the inferior oblique muscle in v-pattern exotropia. *Arch. Ophthalmol.*, 82:21,1969
3. Brown H.W.: Vertical deviations. In symposium strabismus: *Trans Am. Acad. Ophthalmol. Otolaryngol.*, 57: 157, 1963.
4. Eugene R.F.: Strabismus: *Principles and Practice of Ophthalmology*, vol.3, Gholam A. P. et al (EDS), Phidelphia, W.B. Saunders Co, 1st Indian edn., 1987.
5. Fink W.H.: The A and V. syndrome. *Am. Orthopt. J.*, 9: 105, 1959.
6. Gobin M.H.: Sagittalisation of the oblique muscles as possible cause for the A and V and X phenomena. *Br. J. Ophthalmol.*, 52: 13, 1968.
7. Knapp P: A and V pattern, In *Symposium on strabismus: Trans. New Orleans Academy of Ophthalmology.* St. Louis, C.V. Mosby, 1971.
8. Lyle and Jackson's *Practical Orthoptics in the Treatment of Squint*, 5th edn. H.K. Lewis & Co., London, 1967 .
9. Miller J.E.: Vertical recti transplantation in the A and V syndrome. *Arch. Ophthalmol.*, 64:175, 1960
10. Noorden Gunter K.V.: *Binocular Vision and Ocular Motility*, 4th edn. St. Louis, C.V. Mosby Co., 1990.
11. Parks M.M.: The weakening surgical procedure for eliminating overaction of the inferior oblique muscle. *Am. J. Ophthalmol.*, 75:107, 1972.

12. Stanworth A.: A and V syndrome. *Br. J. Orthopt.*, 26:12- 28,1969.
13. Urist M.J: Horizontal squint with secondary vertical deviation. *Arch. Ophthalmol.*, 46: 245, 1951.
14. Urist M.J.: Surgical treatment of esotropia with bilateral elevation in adduction. *Arch. Ophthalmol.*,47: 270,1952.
15. Urist M.J.: The etiology of the so-called A and V syndrome. *Am. J. Ophthalmol.*, 46: 835, 1958.
16. Urist M.J.: Recession and upward displacement of the medial rectus in A pattern exotropia. *Am. J. Ophthalmol.*, 65: 765, 1968.
17. Villaseca A.: The A and V syndrome. *Am. J. Ophthalmol.*, 52: 172, 1961.
18. Shin G.S., Elliot R.L. et al: *J. Pediatric Ophth.*, Sep/Oct 96, 33(5), pp. 211-18.
19. Forster W. Lainch et al: Unilateral tucking and advancement of inferior oblique muscle for treatment of A-pattern strabismus. Klin Monatsbi Angenheiled (German) Nov 1995, 207/5 pp. 305-9. (Medline Indexing Data – 9605, ISSN 0023-2165, Lengnage – German – Unique NLM Identifier 9613 to 29).

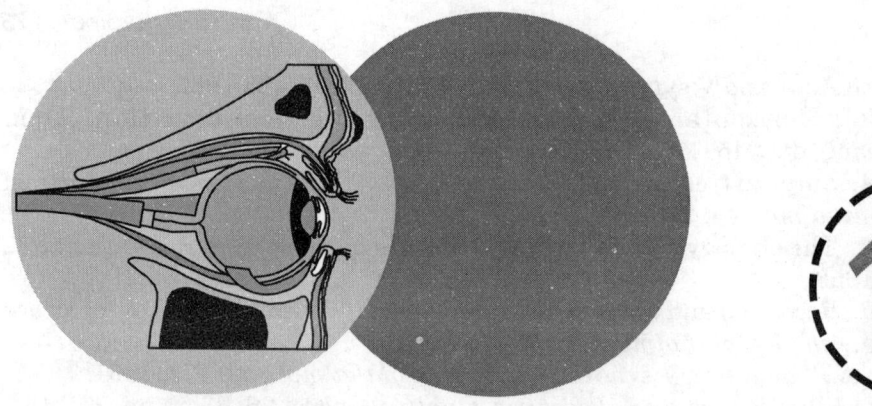

Vertical Squint

The diagnosis and management of vertical strabismus need special care as there are many facts and certain features which still elude explanation. Bielsckowsky[1] in 1938 classified these deviations into five groups.

1. Purely concomitant vertical deviations or hypertropia.
2. Paralytic vertical deviations.
3. Dissociated vertical deviations (DVD).
4. Deviations with unilateral overaction of inferior oblique muscle.
5. Vertical deviations associated with mechanical factors (endocrine myopathy, orbital floor fracture, etc.)

Concomitant Vertical Deviations

Of these purely concomitant vertical deviations (the primary type) are not common. To find a patient with a significant vertical deviation of the same magnitude in all positions of gaze with either eye fixating is unusual.

Following are of the characteristic features of these concomitant vertical deviations (Von Noorden[8]).

1. The deviation is generally smaller in magnitude.
2. Sensory adaptations like amblyopia and abnormal retinal correspondence [ARC] are less frequent since most of these cases are intermittent in nature.
3. Those deviations which are of permanent nature may be associated with a compensatory tilting of the head towards the side of hypotropic eye to

counterbalance the vertical displacement of the images in the two eyes and bring them to the same level.

4. Hyperdeviation of only 2 Δ to 3 Δ prism dioptre can cause headache, eye strain, diplopia or blurred vision, specially in cases of intermittent type wherein the fusional ability) which is sufficiently strong to maintain the visual axis in alignment, may fail under abnormal demand.

Etiology

The etiology of a true concomitant vertical squint is not clear. Some of the cases start as a paretic deviation, which with the passage of time acquired a concomitant look. In others, it was inferior oblique muscle overaction with a concomitant convergent strabismus. In a few, it has been caused by anatomical or mechanical factors of abnormal innervation. As far as anatomical factors are concerned, one may refer to the asymmetry of the orbit or displacement of the globe by a space-occupying lesion. Again, the anatomy of the vertical muscle may be anomalous, causing an imbalance between the elevator and depressor muscles from variations in their insertions, or presence of abnormal attachments and bands.

Treatment

In cases of vertical squint, the treatment is generally surgical, though in some cases, the use of prism with base up and down may temporarily help to relieve the symptoms (Duke–Elder)[2]. In those cases where the vertical deviation is less (upto 10 Δ to 12 Δ prism dioptre), lowering the horizontal muscle insertions of the hypertropic eye or raising the insertions of the hypotropic eye may help. In some of these cases, associated with long standing horizontal deviation, the horizontal muscle is dealt with first and this with the passage of time may be enough to eliminate the vertical component of deviation.

But in those where the deviation is purely vertical in nature, operative interference has to take care of the superior/inferior rectus muscle keeping in mind that postoperative insufficiency in elevation is relatively unimportant compared to inadequate depression.

Dissociated Vertical Deviation (DVD)

Dissociated vertical deviation (Figs 13.1 A & B, 13.2) or alternating sursumduction, dissociated vertical divergence, or alternating hypertropia/hyperphoria. This is an anomaly in which dissociation as by covering an eye causes the covered eye to deviate markedly upwards under the cover, and as soon as the cover is removed, the elevated eye comes down and while doing so it may shoot further down to become hypotropic before coming back to normal horizontal alignment with the fellow eye after a few seconds.

It may occur as an isolated phenomenon in patients in whom binocular functions are normal, but is found more often in association with esotropia, (specially infantile esotropia), or exotropia (Helveston[5]).

The anomaly may not give rise to any subjective symptoms. It may be a chance finding that one eye may show an intermittent vertical deviation upwards. This may occur at variable intervals or may be seen in the eyes alternatively, hence it is also knows as alternating hypertropia/hyoperphoria (Fig. 13.1). In some cases frequent elevation may cause subjective symptoms like blurred vision, difficulty in focussing or headache.

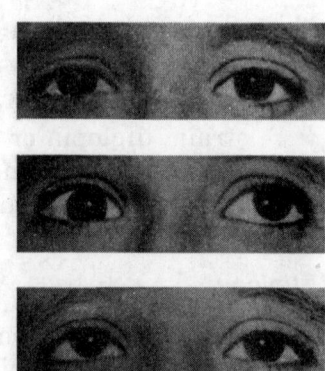

Fig. 13.1 A: Dissociated vertical deviation (DVD)/ alternating hypertropia. Upper figure shows straight eyes; lower figure shows right hypertropia with left eye fixing; middle figure shows left hypertropia with right eye fixing. Photographs taken immediately after the cover was removed from left and right eye.

Etiology

Etiology of DVD is obscure. Various theories have been put forward to explain this condition like (Lyle)[7].

a. The condition is due to a physiological abnormality and is an exaggeration of the normal tendency for the eyes to deviate upwards when they are dissociated by years of occlusion.

b. The condition is due to a pathological disturbance of the uniocular optometer reflexes.

c. The underlying cause is an ocular palsy due to bilateral paresis of the depressor muscles, either the superior oblique or the inferior rectus or both.

The last factor thus divides such cases of dissociated vertical deviation into two groups (Lyle)[7] paralytic and non-paralytic. The paralytic cases may show some evidence of the presence of a paresis in a compensatory head posture (CHP), an adaptation which secures binocular single vision.

Examination of the cases of alternating hypertropia or DVD:

1. Cover test: The covered eye slowly deviates upwards to a variable extent. On removal of the cover, there is a recovery movement downwards which occasionally may be excessive before the final movement to gain fixation. Each eye may show such a updrift under cover.

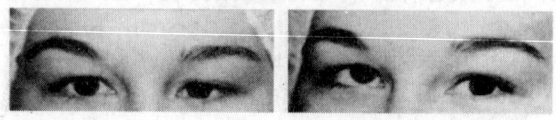

Fig. 13.1 B: Left hypotropia with right eye fixing. Right hypertropia with left eye fixing.

2. Ocular movements Such cases (the paralytic ones) may show a defect of elevation or depression of one or both eyes in one of the oblique positions accompanied by a corresponding overaction of the synergic muscle of the other eye.

3. Since a number of such cases coexist with esotropia/exotropia, mostly infantile esotropia- binocular function is defective in these cases. Others with no horizontal deviation may show normal binocular single vision although there is a strong tendency for suppression.

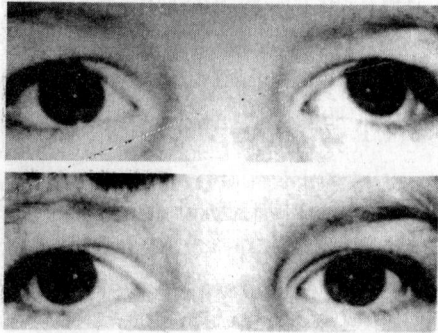

Fig. 13.2: *A case of alternating hyper-tropia. Left-sided hypertropia in upper figure and right-sided hypertropia in lower figure.*

4. In those with poor binocular single vision an increasing head tilt towards the shoulder on the side of the fixing eye and decreasing on tilting the head towards the shoulder on the side of the non-fixing eye may be seen. The non-fixing eye is hypertropic.

5. Diplopia In some cases it may be complained of specially in those with manifest horizontal deviation.

Differential Diagnosis

It may be necessary to differentiate cases of horizontal concomitant deviation with up-shoot of the inferior oblique muscle in adduction from cases of alternating hypertropia. In the latter case, the covered eye becomes elevated in abduction, primary position and adduction, whereas in those with inferior oblique overaction, the eye becomes elevated primarily in adduction and never in abduction. This is obvious and covering of the eye may not be necessary (Noorden)[8]

Treatment

As patients with DVD usually are asymptomatic, the upshoot of the eye under cover may not pose any problem but when the patient is conscious and cosmetically disturbed, surgical correction has to be taken recourse to. This may be a recession of the superior rectus muscle or a combined recession of the superior rectus and recession of the inferior oblique muscle (Knapp)[6].

In the nonparalytic group where there is an association of alternating convergent squint or a constant divergent sign, the treatment is mostly surgical. In such cases correction of the horizontal deviation may appear to lessen the frequency and degree of vertical deviation. Later on, where necessary bilateral superior rectus recession may be necessary to reduce the extent of the vertical deviation.

Vertical Deviation with Overaction of the Inferior Oblique Muscle (Strabismus Sursoaductorious)

A clinical condition in which one finds a marked upshoot of the eye as it moves inwards or adducts. This has been called strabismus sursoadductorious. There is left hypertropia when the eyes deviate to up and right position (dextroversion) and right hypertropia when the eyes in conjugate movement move up and left (laevoversion). In the primary position looking straight ahead, there is no vertical deviation. This condition may be unilateral or bilateral.

It may be an isolated phenomenon when associated with esotropia, mostly congenital esotropia. It may be assumed that in the adducted eye (esotropic eye) the inferior oblique muscle (being a stronger muscle than its counterpart the superior oblique) has a mechanical advantage and the adducted eye shoots up.

But no such explanation is available to explain the upshoot of the inferior oblique in cases where there is no esotropia or paresis/paralysis of the ipsilateral superior oblique or contralateral superior rectus.

Strabismus sarsoadductorious is better left alone for it is not much of a cosmetic problem. Surgery is indicated on occasion when the hypertropia produced by the overacting inferior oblique muscle presents an obstruction to fusion in lateral gaze or a V pattern exists.

Guibor[3] suggested that the possible non-surgical treatment be attempted before operating the inferior oblique muscle.

Cases other than concomitant hypertropia/hyperphoria — Cases of non-comitant vertical deviations are more commonly seen.

They may be broadly grouped into (1) primary vertical strabismus, and (2) secondary vertical strabismus (Villaseca, 1955, quoted by Lyle[7]).

In the primary non-comitant group, we may have cases of.

1. Paresis of an elevator or depressor of one eye.
2. Paralysis of both elevators or depressors of one eye.
3. Bilateral paralysis of the same muscle in each eye.
4. Mixed or multiple paresis—paresis of an elevator of one eye and a depressor of the other eye.

If a purely vertical deviation which was originally latent becomes manifest in childhood due to decompensation, it will tend to be accompanied by a convergent squint because of the strong power of convergence present. If, however, exophoria existed previously, the accompanying horizontal deviation may be divergent.

The Secondary Vertical Strabismus

A typical example is when there is elevation in adduction in a case of convergent squint brought about by the overaction of ipsilateral inferior oblique. This is the concomitant type which has already been mentioned earlier. The secondary variety of non-comitant type of inferior oblique overaction is caused by paresis or paralysis of the antagonist such as superior oblique muscle in the same eye or contralateral synergist, the superior rectus in the other eye. Cases of A and V syndrome can also be cited as cases of secondary vertical strabismus wherein as a result of the relative strength in adduction/abduction, cases of convergent/divergent horizontal strabismus tend to have elevation/depression in certain positions of gaze.

In primary vertical squints the horizontal deviation does not vary whether the gaze is directed straight up, straight ahead or straight down whereas horizontal deviation varies in a case of horizontal squint with a secondary vertical component.

A compensatory head posture is evident in cases of primary non-comitant vertical squint whereas this is not shown in a secondary vertical squint.

Treatment

Treatment of vertical squints is largely a surgical problem. In secondary cases, correction of the horizontal deviation is all that may be necessary—the vertical component disappearing after some time. In primary non-comitant vertical squint cases, operation may have to be done on both horizontal and vertical muscles at the same time. Some prefer to operate on horizontal first and the vertical muscle is taken care in the second sitting.

Primary Vertical Strabismus

The details of the *primary group* are described in Chapter 14. However, one would like to mention about superior oblique palsy, and double elevator palsy, for they frequently creep in while discussing hyper deviation cases.

The superior oblique is the only vertical muscle that has its innervation from a single nerve (the trochlear nerve) and as such the most common paretic hyperdeviation results from a palsy of the fourth cranial nerve and superior oblique muscle.

The amount of vertical deviation is greater in the early onset cases and less in the acquired ones. Traumatic cases complain of diplopia. The most common symptom or complaint in congenital cases is the position of one eye being higher than the other and an unsightly head tilt.

Double elevator palsy is a common cause of hyperdeviation. Examination reveals a paresis of the superior rectus and inferior oblique muscles both in the same eye. Ptosis may be an associated finding. The child generally walks with the head elevated slightly to maintain binocular single vision.

An occasional association in such cases may be Marcus-Gunn jaw-winking phenomenon.

The etiology is difficult to explain and the treatment is surgical correction, though seldom indicated, for a number of such cases have binocular single vision in the primary straight ahead position and are aware of diplopia only on looking up.

Complete Third Nerve Palsy

A patient with complete third nerve palsy may show a hyperdeviation, though this is rare. Hyperdeviation results when of the muscles supplied by the nerve, not all but a few show weakness or paresis. An example being paresis of the superior rectus (the other muscles having recovered from paresis or paralysis) supplied by the upper division of the third nerve.

Special Group

There is a special group situation in which a patient may have a vertical deviation caused by an orbital condition like thyroid myopathy. The patient cannot elevate the eye above the midline in the field of action of the super rectus. The condition is bilateral though to start with there may be gross assymetry. Some of these cases may also show esotropia or limitation of movement in adduction (abduction/ elevation).

The pathology is perhaps due to fibrosis of the extraocular muscles, inferior, superior and/or medical rectus. Of these fibrosis of the inferior rectus is more common. At times the inferior rectus is just a tight band that can actually indent the sclera.

Blow-out Fracture

As a result of blunt injury to the eye, the orbital floor gives way. The inferior rectus and occasionally the inferior oblique are trapped in the fracture. Limitation of the action of the superior and inferior rectus and occasionally of the inferior oblique results. There may also be relative enophthalmos (see Chapter 15 for details).

The eye may be straight in the primary position or the patient may have a hypertropia with diplopia in the up and down position.

REFERENCES

1. Bielschowksy A.: Disturbances of the vertical motor muscles of the eye. *Arch. Ophthalmol*, 20:175,1938.
2. Duke-Elder, S. and Wybar K: *System of Ophthalmology*, vol.6.: *Ocular Motility and Strabismus.* St. Louis, The C V Mosby Co., 1973.
3. Guibor G.P.: Synkinetic overaction of the inferior oblique muscle. *Am. J. Ophthalmol.*, 22:100, 1949.

4. Edward W., Cheeseman J., David L., Guyton M. D.: Vertical fusional vergence — the key to dissociated vertical deviation. *Arch Ophthalmol,* 117: 1188 1999 (Sept.).

5. Helveston E.M.: Dissociated vertical deviation – A clinical and laboratory study. *Trans Am. Ophthalmic Soc.,* 78:734, 1980.

6. Knapp, P.: Dissociated vertical deviation, in Fells P. (Editor): *Proc. Second Congress International Strabismological Association,* Marseilles, 1976.

7. Lyle T. K. and Wybar K.: *Practical Orthoptics in the Treatment of Squint,* London, H.K. Lewis and Co., 1967.

8. Noorden G.K.: *Binocular Vision and Ocular Motility — Theory and Management of Strabismus,* 3rd edn. St. Louis, The C.V. Mosby Co., 1985.

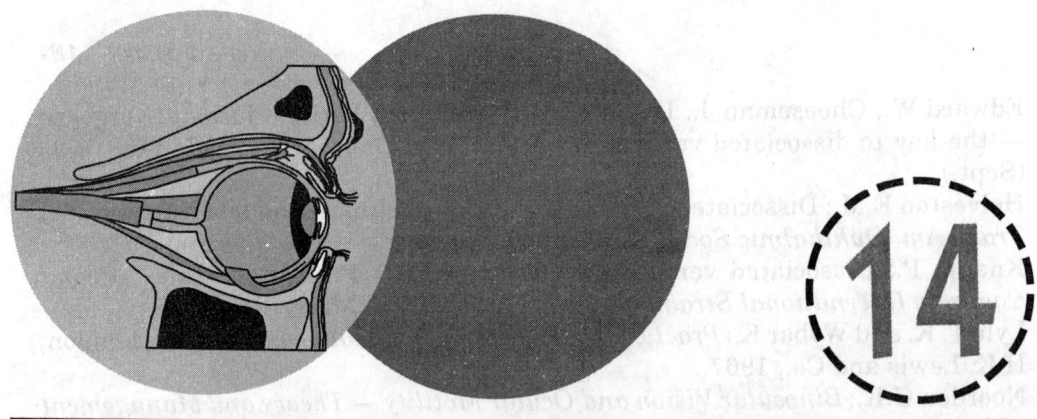

Paralytic Squint

A dissociation of ocular movements wherein, the deviation is irregular and varies in an uncoordinated manner (in different directions of the gaze) results in a paralytic or noncomitant squint. Such a squint or deviation becomes evident when the eye is turned in a way that the affected muscle comes into play. It becomes more pronounced, the further the eye is moved in this direction; on the other hand it may not ordinarily be evident in movements in which the affected muscle does not participate.

Diagnosis of a recent onset ocular muscle paresis/paralysis is not particularly difficult. The patient is disturbed by double-vision or diplopia which increases in intensity as the eye is turned in the direction of the paretic or paralysed muscle. On the other hand, diagnosis of a congenital or a long standing paresis/paralysis can present a formidable clinical challenge. The clinical picture may change significantly within weeks after the onset of paresis or paralysis.

The first stage is characterised by the weakness of the paralysed muscle. This is followed as a rule by overaction of its direct antagonist (ipsilateral). Thus, paralysis of right lateral rectus muscle leads to overaction of the right medial rectus muscle (Fig. 14.1). The contralateral synergist medial rectus of the other eye (left eye in the present case) undergoes overaction.

As per Hering's law of equal innervation there is an equal distribution of innervational impulses between the two eyes and as a consequence of greater effort put forward to move the paralysed muscle (right lateral rectus in the present case) there is a compensatory spasm of the contra-lateral associate of the paretic muscle the contralateral synergist, the left medial rectus muscle.

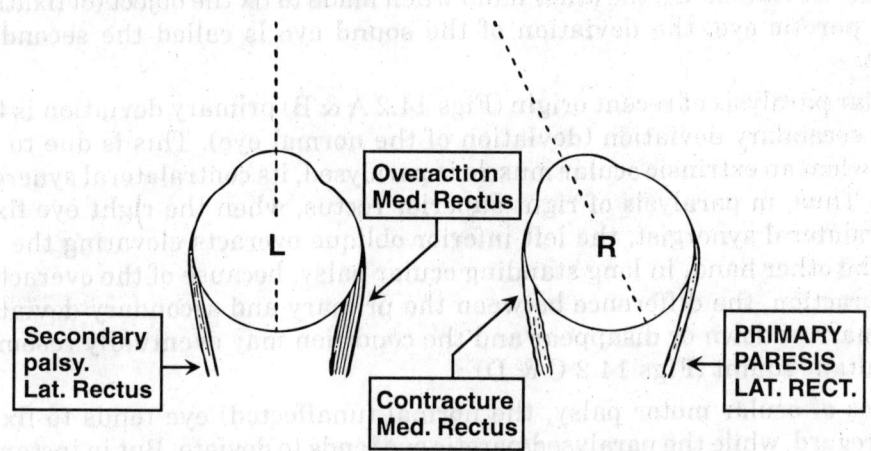

1. PARESIS OF R. LAT. RECTUS

Overaction
Med. Rectus

L   R

Secondary
palsy.
Lat. Rectus

Contracture
Med. Rectus

PRIMARY
PARESIS
LAT. RECT.

Fig. 14.1:   Paresis of right lateral rectus with overaction of direct antagonist and subsequent changes in medial and lateral rectus in left eye.

And this in turn leads to a secondary inhibitional plasy of the contralateral anatogonist[3], the left lateral rectus.

In course of time these contractures, overaction and underation may lead to the original noncomitant squint becoming virtually concomitant.

Symptomatology

Diplopia is the main symptom which unnerves the patient. It is more pronounced in recent cases. In untreated and long standing cases, it may gradually be overcome by suppression of the image from the paralytic eye or as a result of compensatory head posture (CHP) developing, it may not be felt in the primary straight-ahead position of the eye.

Examination and Investigation

An abnormal deviation of the eye is evident in the primary straight ahead-position of the eye. It is more marked when a vertical muscle is paralysed. The direction of the deviation depends on the muscle paralysed. Thus, in paralysis of right lateral rectus, the right eye fails to make movements outwards to the right (dextrodeviation). On the other hand, in paresis/paralysis of long standing, the picture may change as already mentioned.

Deviation Demonstration: Cover Test

While doing a cover test, a patient with paralysis of an extrinsic ocular muscle prefers to fix the target object with the sound (unaffected) eye while the affected paralysed eye undergoes deviation. This deviation of the paralysed eye is called the primary deviation. On the other hand when made to fix the object (of fixation) with his paretic eye, the deviation of the sound eye is called the secondary deviation.

In ocular paralysis of recent origin (Figs 14.2 A & B) primary deviation is less than the secondary deviation (deviation of the normal eye). This is due to the fact that when an extrinsic ocular muscle is paralysed, its contralateral synergist overacts. Thus, in paralysis of right superior rectus, when the right eye fixes, the contralateral synergist, the left inferior oblique overacts elevating the left eye. On the other hand, in long standing ocular palsy, because of the overaction and underaction, the difference between the primary and secondary deviation tends to narrow down or disappear and the condition may eventually resemble a concomitant squint (Figs 14.2 C & D)..

In cases of ocular motor palsy, the normal (unaffected) eye tends to fix an object of regard, while the paralysed/paretic eye tends to deviate. But in instances as described below, the paralysed eye may tend to fix.

1. When the paretic eye has better vision and it has been the master eye, and/or

2. When while fixing with paralysed eye, diplopia is less troublesome.

Adoption of Compensatory Postural Attitude

To overcome diplopia and consequent confusion, the patient tends to assume a postural attitude in which the paretic muscle is sufficiently relieved of its function, whereby the diplopia is least marked and/or binocular single vision is possible. It is a functional adaptation to abolish or lessen diplopia. It has three components: (1) rotation of face, (2) head tilting, and (3) elevation or depression of the chin.

Rotation of face The face is turned in the direction in which the diplopia is greatest, that is, in the direction of the field of action of the paralysed muscle. Thus, in a case of right lateral rectus palsy, the face is turned to right so that the eyes are looking to the left (laevoversion) relative to the orbital axis. This relaxes the right lateral muscle, the paralysed muscle.

In paresis of an elevator: The greatest separation of the image occurs when the eyes are raised and least when they are lowered. Thus, in paresis of superior rectus and inferior oblique (both elevators) the face is raised with the chin elevated, so that a downward position of the eye is encouraged to minimise the diplopia. The reverse is seen with paralysis of inferior rectus and superior oblique (the depressor muscles).

Since the superior and inferior recti have their greatest vertical effectivity on abduction, the vertical deviation becomes progressively less when the affected eye is adducted for in this position the vertical component of the recti becomes less effective and that of obliques more effective. And to allow for adduction of

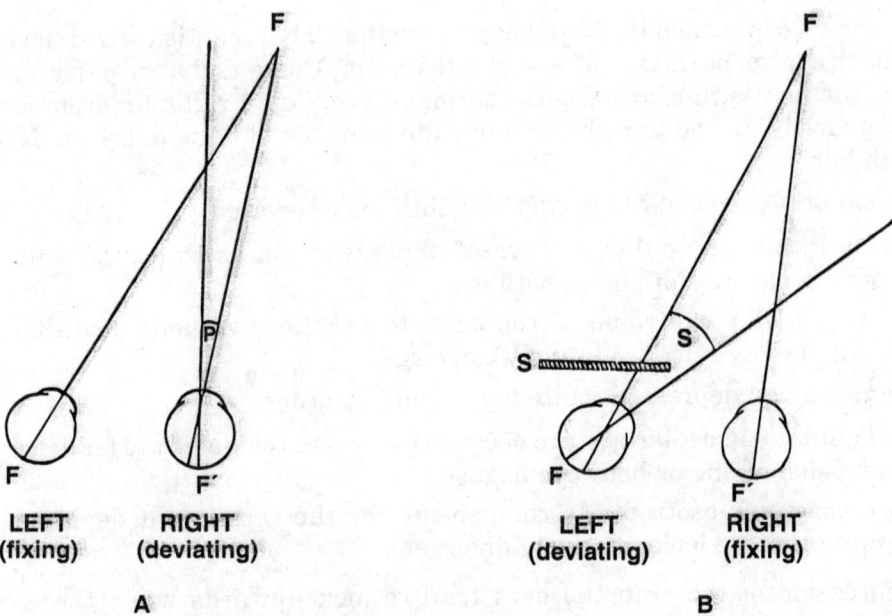

LEFT (fixing) **RIGHT** (deviating)

A

LEFT (deviating) **RIGHT** (fixing)

B

Fig. 14.2 A & B: In a recent paralytic squint affecting the right eye, the primary deviation P in (A) is less than the secondary S in (B) obtained when the non-squinting normal eye is covered by a screen s.

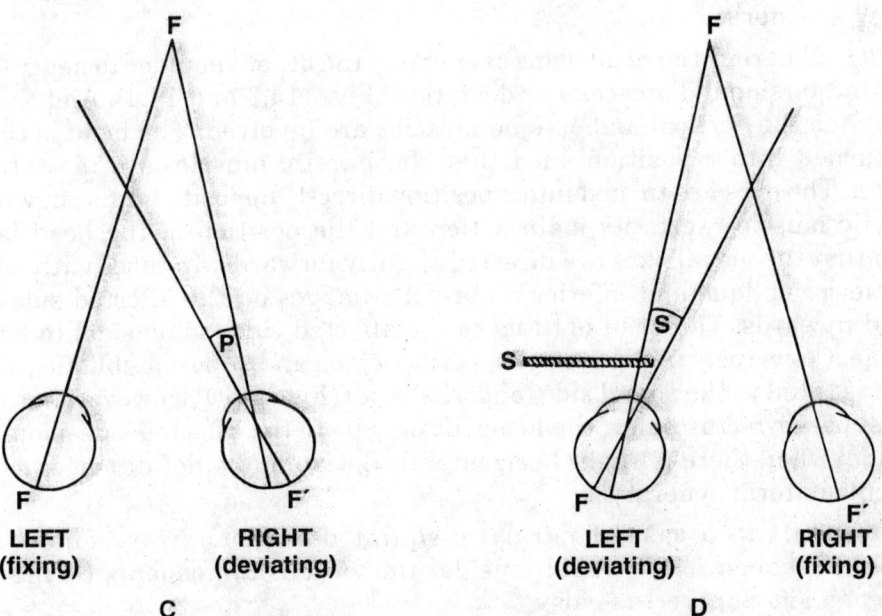

LEFT (fixing) **RIGHT** (deviating)

C

LEFT (deviating) **RIGHT** (fixing)

D

Fig. 14.2 C & D: In concomitant squint (affecting the right eye) the primary deviation P (A) is equal to the secondary deviation S (B) obtained when the nonsquinting eye is occluded by a screen s.

the eye, the face is turned in the opposite direction. That is, it is turned towards the palsied eye in paralysis of a vertical rectus. Conversely, in palsy of the obliques, the face is turned towards the sound eye, i.e. in right superior rectus palsy, the face is turned to right, and in right superior oblique palsy the face is turned to left.

Elevation or depression of the chin The chin may elevated

1. To maintain an ocular posture of depression so as to compensate for defective elevator of one or both eye.
2. In a case of V-exotropia to compensate for the divergent deviation by making the eyes look relatively convergent.

While it may be depressed (chin-depression) in order.

i. To maintain an ocular posture of elevation so as to compensate for defective depression of one or both eye as also
ii. In a case of V-esotropia to compensate for the convergent deviation by making the eye look relatively divergent.

In depression of the chin the eyes tend to look upwards when there is a tendency to diverge slightly, which is the physiological phenomenon.

On the other hand elevation of the chin causes the eyes to look downward and with this is associated the physiological activity of increased convergence and this may overcome a slight degree of exotropia or relieve the symptoms caused by exophoria.

Head tilt Whereby the head leans over one or the other shoulder to neutralise vertical and torsional displacement/deviation (Figs. 14.3 and 14.4). And this is evident when the vertical and oblique muscles are involved. The head is tilted and/or turned into a position such that the paretic muscle is in a state of relaxation. The eyes are turned into a position directly opposite to that in which the paretic muscle exerts its main action and the position of the head is so adjusted that the visual axes are directed slightly forwards. In cases with palsy of the inferior oblique and inferior rectus, the images on the affected side are displaced upwards. The head is tilted to the affected side (same side) to lower this image. Conversely in the case of superior rectus and superior oblique palsy, the head is tilted to the sound side (opposite side) (Fig. 14.4). However, in cases of right superior rectus palsy, the head tilt may be to the affected side shoulder (same side) when there is slight horizontal deviation and a definite overaction of the contralateral synergist.

The head-tilt in a case of paralytic squint does not always follow the physiological sequence. We would consider the various components taking the example of a left Sup. rectus palsy.

1. Position of the head to correct the vertical deviation: Since the left superior rectus (LSR) is an elevator, its paralysis would cause the eyes to go down relatively and to chin being elevated. As the left SR is a left-hand elevator,

R   L

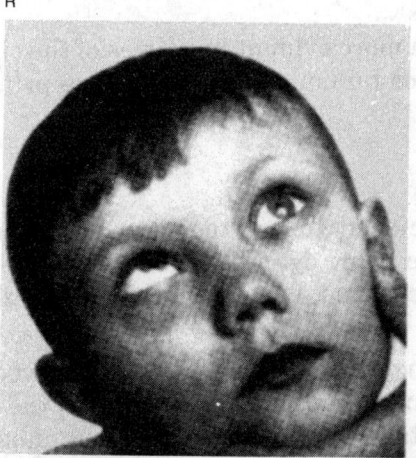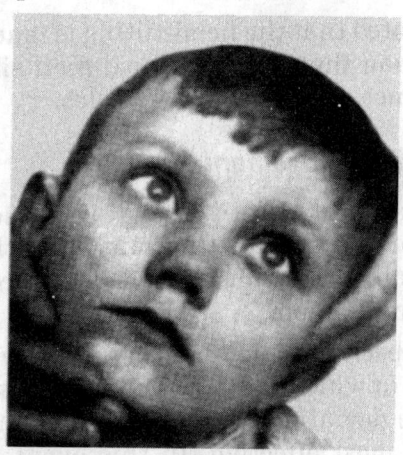

Fig. 14.3: Compensatory head posture. A patient with right superior oblique palsy the head it tilted to left shoulder and the face is slightly turned to the left. Right hypertropia increases on tilting the head to the paralysed side (right) while in right superior rectus palsy the right eye goes down (hypotropia) or shows no change in position on tilting to the paralysed right side.

it will be desirable to turn the eyes not only downward but also to the right to reduce the vertical deviation still more. Hence not only is the chin raised but the face is turned to the left. The face is turned up and to the left; the eyes are turned away from the position of maximum vertical action of the paralysed left superior rectus.

2. Position of the head to correct the horizontal deviation: LSR is an adductor, hence its palsy may cause exotropia (causing horizontal separation of the image) which would increase by turning the eye to the right, same as turning the head to the left. Hence, when exotropia is pronounced the head may be turned to the right. On the other hand when there is no separation of the images, there may be little or no lateral turning of the head.

3. Position of the head to correct torsion: With LSR palsy the eyeball is not only rotated down and out (by overacting LIR) but the vertical corneal meridian is extorted by overacting LIO. To correct or compensate for this extorsion, the head may be tiled sideway towards the right side. But it must be understood that head tilting may not be always adopted strictly as analysed above.

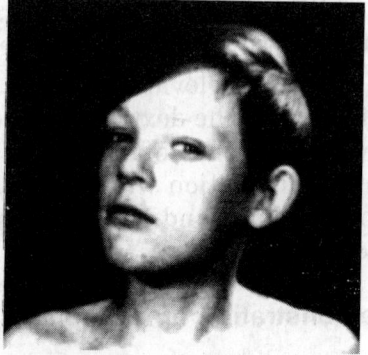

Fig. 14.4: A patient of right superior rectus palsy with the tilting of the head towards the shoulder of the sound side (left); please note that in such a case of some duration this will usually be masked by a tilt towards the shoulder of the paralysed side (right).

Be it noted that the head-tilting is much more evident in palsies of the oblique muscle than that of the vertical recti since torsions of the globe are primarily the province of the oblique muscles.

Limitation of Movement

The muscles of the two eyes are associated to act together in conjugate movements: The adducting muscle of the right eye (RMR), for example, acts with the abducting muscle (left lateral rectus) as if they constitute a single left handed mechanism.

On inspection little abnormality may be evident if the eyes are moved in a direction in which the affected muscle is not an important factor. On the other hand, the deviation would be greater in that direction in which the muscle is normally most effective. In this event, in paralysis the affected eye will lag behind the normal and will eventually come to a standstill while the normal eye completes its exercise, while in spasm it would overshoot the other.

Limitation of movement is less noticeable in paralysis of vertical recti and least in paralysis of the obliques but it is usually demonstrable if the conjugate ocular movements are carefully examined and the excursion of the two eyes are compared.

With the vertical muscles, it has to be understood that the greatest vertical pull each muscle is capable of exerting is only when the eyeball is in certain position. Thus the LSR/left superior rectus) rotates the eyeball up and in from the primary straight-ahead position but the greatest vertical deviation of the eye is obtained by this muscle (LSR) only when the eyeball is rotated to the left, the LSR being a laevoelevator. Right inferior oblique is the other laevoelevator and the two muscles work to elevate the eyeball up and to the left.

The dextroelevator or right hand elevators are right superior recti and left inf oblique. The dextrodepressors or right hand depressor are the right inferior rectus and the left superior oblique. These muscles exert their maximal depressing action when the eyeballs are in a position of rotation to the right. And the left hand laevodepressors are right superior oblique and left inferior rectus.

Demonstration of Diplopia

Demonstrating the presence and type of diplopia is a useful guide in diagnosis of paralytic squint. It is helpful in pointing out the muscle or muscles involved in the paresis/paralysis.

Diplopia Test

Armstrong[4] *bar-lite* along with a red and white glass is used for the diplopia test (Fig. 14.5). The patient (with right rectus palsy for example) should be seated keeping, his head perfectly still and erect throughout the investigation.

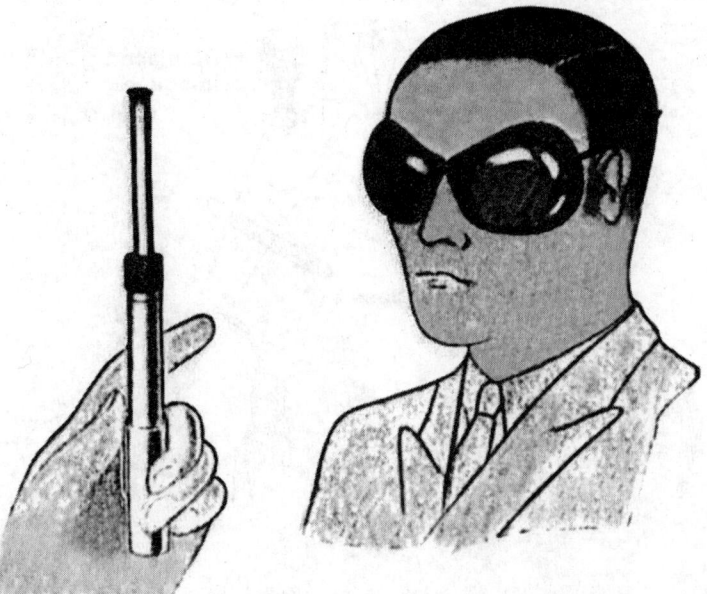

Fig. 14.5:   Armstrong bar-light and goggles for the investigation of diplopia.

At a distance of one meter in front of the patient, the examiner holds the source of light. The Armstrong barlite gives a rod of light 1.5 inches long. The patient puts on the goggles with the red glass in front of the right eye and looks at the light (Fig. 14.6). If two images are present, one red and the other white, the red has been seen through the right eye (with red glass in front of it). The light is then moved to the right and to the left, then up and down and up and out to left, up and out to right, and down and out to the left, and finally down and out to the right.

The position in which the diplopia appears and in which the separation of the images is most marked is noted (Fig. 14.6). The distal image belongs to the paralysed eye.

With the lateral muscles, the diplopia is horizontal and with vertical muscles it is vertically separated. In addition, in oblique muscles, the image may be tilted as a result of torsional deviation.

Diplopia Chart

Giving the images in cases of paralysis of extrinsic ocular muscles (Fig. 14.7) for right lateral rectus palsy and Fig. 14.8 for right superior oblique palsy.

Measurement on the Synoptophore

Precise information and measurement of the horizontal, vertical and torsional deviation in the cardinal directions of the eye movement with each eye fixing in

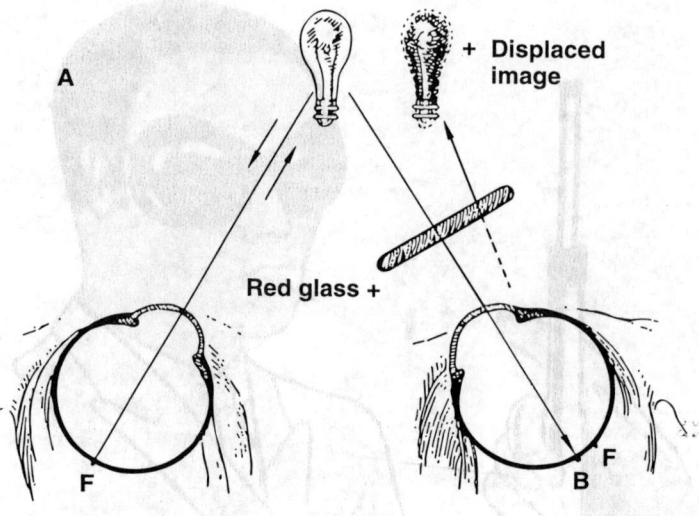

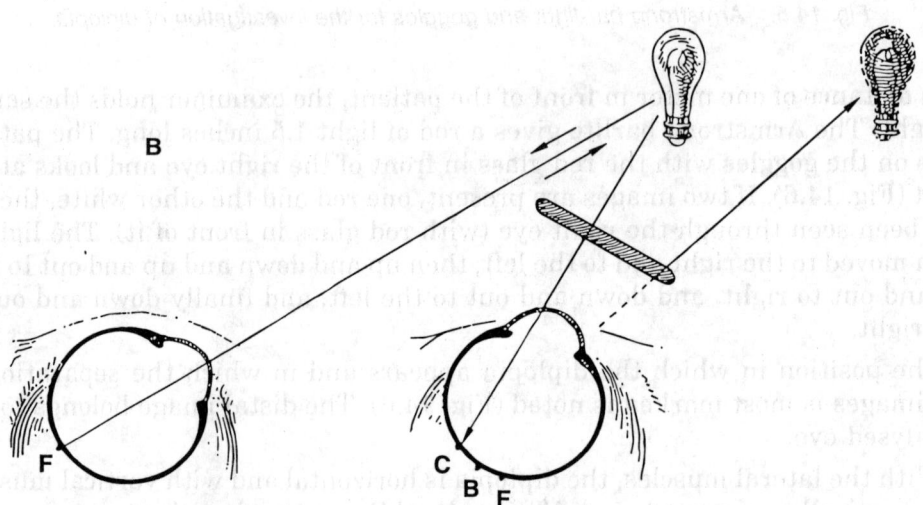

Fig. 14.6: *A patient with right lateral rectus palsy — use of a goggle with red glass in front of the right eye and a plane white glass in front of the left eye along with Armstrong bar light. This demonstrates diplopia and its nature.*

turn can be made upto 15° from the mid-plane. These measurements can be made both objectively and subjectively. The information so obtained is useful when planning operative-treatment and when assessing the results of such treatment.

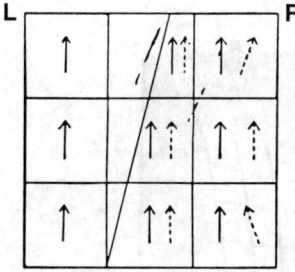

Fig. 14.7: *Diplopia charting: Right lateral rectus palsy.*

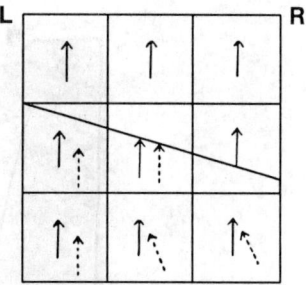

Fig. 14.8: *Diplopia charting: Right superior oblique palsy.*

Screen-test with Red and Green Glasses

Examination on an electrically operated Hess Screen using a red and green glass/goggle and where red spot lights are substituted for red dots on the background screen and a movable illuminated green indicator substituted for the green cord is designed to give a better or more accurate result (Figs 14.9, 14.10 and 14.11). It provides a permanent and accurate record of the deviation, the muscle or muscles involved as also of the secondary changes in the ipsilateral and contralateral antagonist and synergist. Recorded at suitable intervals of time, it provides important data with regard to the progress of the case. The same is now available in computerised form.

Fields of Fixation

The field of uniocular-fixation is that area within which foveal fixation of a small test object can occur, whereas the field of binocular fixation is that area within which bifocal fixation of a small test object can occur. Its extent is limited partly by the limits of the ocular movement and partly by the nose. The extent of the field of binocular fixation can be determined by means of a perimeter. Such recording of the extent (of binocular field of fixation) before and after operation in a case of ocular palsy may give an idea of the recovery or rate of recovery of the ocular palsy. However, this determination of binocular field of fixation is not of much clinical value and hence not commonly employed in clinical practice.

False Orientation or False Projection

In cases of recent paralysis of an extrinsic ocular muscle, when the sound eye is covered and an object is held in various positions in the field of vision and the patient asked to touch the object with the tip of his finger, it is found that he points beyond the object (past-pointing) when the latter is situated in the field governed by the paretic muscle. The explanation of the fact is that the patient

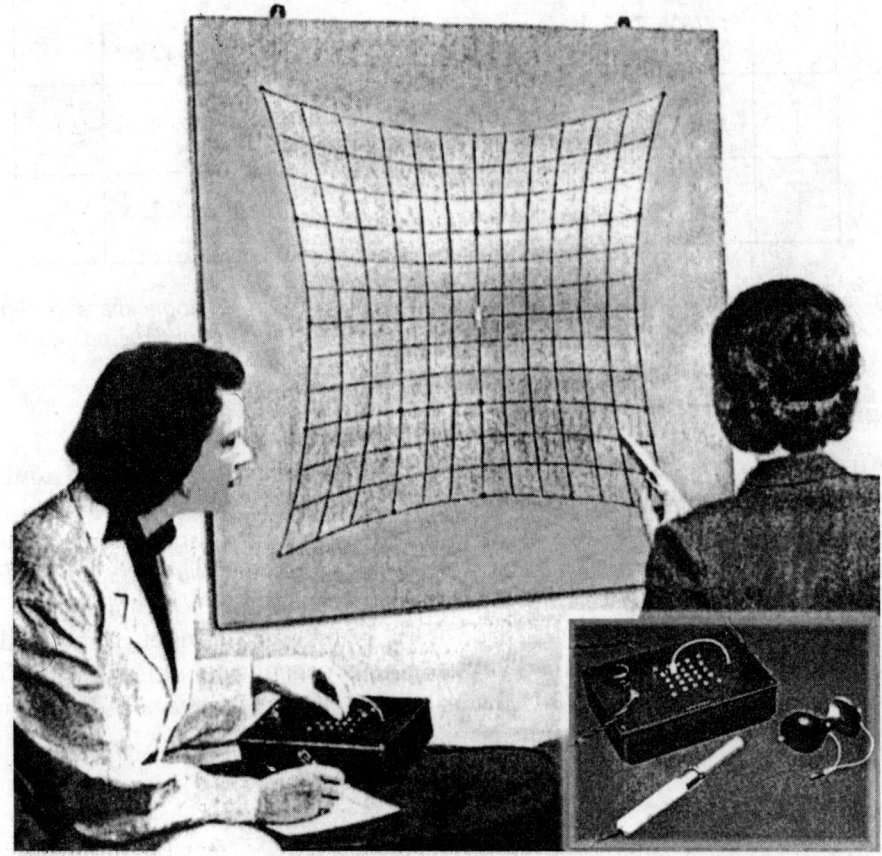

Fig. 14.9:   *Hess screen electrically operated.*

has to put on extra neuromuscular effort to turn his eyes, so that he estimates the object as farther away than is actually the case.

Etiology

Etiologically, cases of paralytic squint could be divided into two distinct groups (1) congenital paralytic squint, and (2) acquired paralytic squint.

Congenital Paralytic Squint

Such a squint may be constant squint, or a deviation only in certain directions of the gaze, binocular single vision being obtained in other directions of the gaze. The constant type is more likely to occur with one muscle or more paralysed/paresed at birth, there being no evidence as to a possible inflammatory or traumatic cause. Similarly, there is no clarity as to the site of the lesion in or of the nerve supplying the muscle or in the muscle itself.

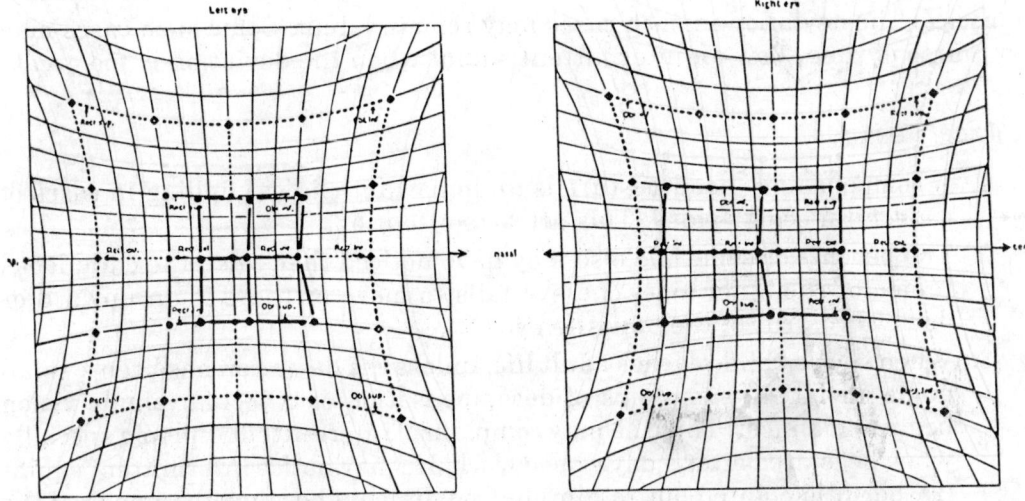

Fig. 14.10: *Hess screen chart in left lateral rectus palsy.*

In some cases of horizontal squint in infants, a careful examination of the ocular muscles may show that there is an underlying vertical muscle palsy which is probably the primary cause of the deviation, the horizontal deviation being secondary.

Cases where the deviation is evident only in certain directions of the gaze and binocular vision is obtainable in other directions of the gaze, show a compensatory head-posture. This avoids the use of the affected muscle or

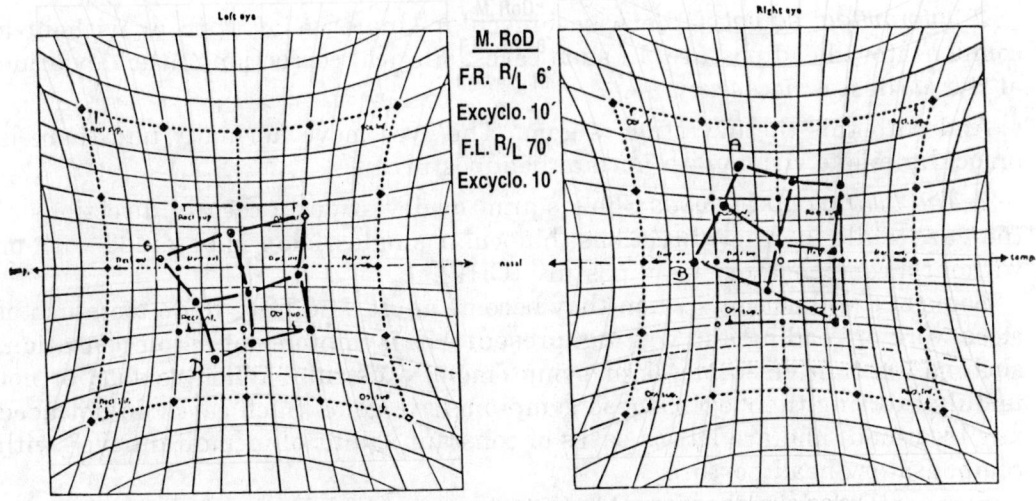

Fig. 14.11: *Hess screen chart in right superior oblique palsy.*

muscles. The deviation in such cases may remain latent. Some such cases may in course of time show an intermittent squint when the deviation is too great.

Clinical Features

1. A compensatory head-posture is an important clinical finding in cases of congenital ocular palsy. This attracts attention.

2. The parents or some one else may have noticed that when the child looks to one or the other side, one eye fails to move or there is an upward or downward drift of the opposite eye.

3. When such a child reaches adult life, unless the deviation has been a small angle deviation, symptoms of decompensation of binocular single vision begin to manifest. Thus, he may complain of intermittent diplopia specially when he is tired after a day's hard work. He may notice intermittent squint (rather it is pointed out to him) but no diplopia because the image of the deviating eye is suppressed. He may find it easier to read with one eye closed (to avoid diplopia). Such cases of congenital ocular palsy have to be differentiated from the cases of acquired ocular palsy[8] (Table 14.1).

Sequence of Events

Cases of congenital ocular paresis/paralysis generally develop along one of the following sequences of events.

1. Constant squint of incomitant type: In these cases, a definite limitation of ocular movement in one or more directions can be seen. Thus, it can be purely horizontal in type or vertical in nature with or without a horizontal component.

2. Intermittent squint: Otherwise binocular single vision with or without a compensatory head posture. In such cases, surgical correction of the deviation at the earliest is necessary.

And with this the deviation is gone, The eyes move normally and there is binocular single vision with normal headposture.

3. The third group of cases Show squint or deviation in certain directions of the gaze while in other directions, binocular single vision is obtained with or without a compensatory head posture (CHP).

Some of these patients when they become adult, and have to do too much of close work or reading and writing, present with symptoms of decompensation, such as intermittent-diplopia or symptoms of eyestrain. When relaxed or not unduly exerting their eyes, these symptoms are gone. Such cases do not need any treatment and are left as cases of constant squint of incomitant type with compensatory head posture.

Some of them do well with orthoptic treatment which improves their binocular function. These cases in particular need operative correction of the deviation.

Table 14.1 Symptoms and Signs in Congenital and Acquired Palsies

Symptoms	Congenital	Acquired
1. Onset of symptom shortly after birth	Usually gradual	Often sudden
2. Age	Usually childhood	Any age
3. Presenting symptoms by the patient himself	i. Intermittent diplopia or diplopia in certain directions of gaze. ii. Difficulty in focussing. iii. Likes to read with one eye closed.	Diplopia in all or only in certain direction of gaze.
4. Signs. i. Head posture.	Compensatory head posture usually present. There is scoliosis.	May occur and the patient is aware of it; no anatomical change in the vertebral column.
ii. Difference between primary and secondary deviation	Generally slight or none, the deviation tends to become concomitant	The characteristic finding of secondary deviation being greater than the primary deviation
iii. Suppression/ARC	Usually present	Suppression absent at first but may occur later
iv. Neurological findings or systemic disease.	Usually absent	May be present

They are thus functionally cured, but may retain some degree of compensatory head posture.

Ocular Torticolis

A compensatory head posture (CHP) associated with congenital ocular palsy usually involves a head tilt, in addition to a face-turn and a raising or lowering of the chin. This may resemble a wry neck or torticollis due to unilateral contracture of the sternocleidomastoid muscle. One likes to call them as cases of ocular torticollis as against the ordinary torticollis.

Table 14.2 shows how an ocular torticollis can be differentiated from an ordinary torticollis.

Table 14.2 Differential Diagnosis of Ordinary and Ocular Torticollis

Ordinary Torticollis	*Ocular Torticollis*
1. Gross contracture of the sterno cleido mastoid muscle on the side of the neck to which the head is tilted. This makes the muscle feel hard on palpation.	1. A slight degree of tightness or stiffness of the structures on the side of the neck to which the head is tilted.
2. Hence the head cannot be passively straightened.	2. Head can be passively straightened, but on so doing the patient is unable to maintain binocular single vision as diplopia is experienced.
3. Face always turned away from the side of the head tilt.	3. The direction in which the face is turned and the position of the chin varies according to the muscle at fault.
4. Conjugate ocular movements normal.	4. Conjugate ocular movement normal/ abnormal.
5. External ocular muscle balance normal.	5. Hypertropia of one eye, with hypotropia of the other eye; the head is tilted towards the hypotropic eye.

Treatment

When considering treatment, cases of congenital paralytic squint can be broadly divided into two groups.

Group 1: Children and young adults in whom binocular single vision is satisfactory as a result of compensatory head posture.

In such cases, treatment aims to sustain the binocular single vision and with normal head posture. And this is possible only by surgical correction of the deviation as early as feasible.

In addition, orthoptic treatment may become necessary after surgery. The general surgical principles would be as follows.

a. To strengthen the action of the weak muscle, or
b. To weaken the overaction of the same-sided (ipsilateral) anatagonistic muscle, or
c. To weaken the overaction of the opposite eye (contralateral) synergistic muscle.
d. To strengthen the underaction of the opposite eye (contralateral) antagonist muscle.

Let us take as example a case of right superior rectus paralysis (congenital) which would be illustrative. Based on the above theoretical principles one may

a. strengthen the right superior rectus, or
b. weaken the right inferior rectus, or
c. weaken the left inferior oblique, or
d. strengthen the left superior oblique.

But of all these, when it comes to surgery, weakening the left inferior oblique, which by its overaction is causing annoying symptoms, is preferable and is the surgery of choice. Weakening the action of inferior rectus muscle which moves the eye downwards would lead to annoying diplopia or discomfort when walking or reading. This is more troublesome to the patient than weakening the action of the inferior oblique muscle (which takes the eye up) for diplopia in this upward movement is easily ignored.

Group 2: The second group is of those cases in which a patient with congenital ocular paralysis has reached the adult life and then starts having symptoms of failure of binocular single vision, namely he notices diplopia when tired after extensive use of the eyes for close-work following some deterioration in the general health. Some of these cases may be relieved of symptoms by temporary use of prismatic lens, however, when symptoms and discomfort persist, operative interference may be necessary.

Acquired Paralytic Squint

Clinical features of an acquired paralytic squint have already been mentioned while differentiating the congenital and acquired paralytic squint. From clinical view point, it would be better to discuss the paralysis of the extraocular muscles individually as also in group.

Etiologically, the cause may be in the muscle, at the neuromuscular junction, in the peripheral nerve in the nuclear region or in the supranuclear ocular pathway. And to elucidate this, the ophthalmologist has to refer his case to a physician, a neurosurgeon and to the diagnostic aids which may include a cat Scan and MRI besides the routine clinical diagnostic aids and examination.

Complete Third Cranial Nerve Palsy

Though not very common, it occasionally poses a challenging thereapeutic problem as most patients are not happy with binocular single vision in the straight ahead position only and eventually may end up using a patch to avoid diplopia.

The partic eye assumes a position of abduction, slight depression and intorsion with a varying degree of ptosis. The lateral rectus and superior oblique are the only two functioning extraocular muscles. With a complete third cranial nerve palsy, the intrinsic muscles of the eye are also involved causing the pupil to be dilated and nonreactive along with paralysis of accommodation.

The motility of the affected eye is limited to abduction and to a small degree of depression and the eye does not move beyond the midline towards adduction.

Common etiological factors are head trauma, raised intra cranial pressure and neoplasm (vascular), diabetes, hypertension and atherosclerosis and supraclinoid aneurysm of internal carotid artery. A large number are, however, undetermined. Paralysis resulting from aneurysm is associated with pain which is sharp and throbbing in character and the pupil on the affected side is dilated and non-reactive. Cases of paralysis from ischaemic causes complain of pain dull and constant in character.

Superior Rectus Palsy

An isolated paralysis of the superior rectus muscle is rare. It is commonly congenital. There is frequently an associated weakness of the homolateral levator palpabrae muscle, particularly when the paralysis is congenital with resulting ptosis. Elevation of the eye is affected and the paralytic eye is hypotropic in primary position.

In paralysis of recent onset, the face is turned upwards, the chin is elevated and the head is usually inclined towards the sound side (shoulder). This leads to the compensatory head posture (CHP), mostly in cases of congenital origin. Fixation with the paretic eye causes hypertropia of the sound eye resulting from overaction of inferior oblique in this sound eye.

Medial Rectus Muscle

An isolated paralysis of the medial rectus is rare. There is restriction of adduction movement of the affected side, e.g. movement of the right eye towards left (adduction) is affected. The patient's face is turned to sound side (left side in the instant case) as a result of the antagonostic lateral rectus overacting.

Inferior Rectus Muscle

An isolated paralysis of the inferior rectus muscle is rare. It may occur following orbital floor trauma, or is congenital. The affected eye's (say the right eye) movement downwards is affected and along with the superior oblique of the other eye (left eye), down and out movement to the right side is also affected. As a result of ipsilateral superior rectus overacting the affected eye is hypertropic in the primary position. A compensatory head posture with the face turn to the paretic side, chin depressed and the head tilting to the same side shoulder is seen (in right inferior rectus paralysis, the CHP is face turned to right, chin depressed and the head tilt commonly to the right shoulder).

Inferior oblique muscle In inferior oblique paralysis the affected eye is hypotropic in the primary position when the patient fixes with the affected eye. On the other hand, when the patient prefers to fix with the sound eye, it is hypertropic. In conjugate movement, the greatest restriction occurs when the eyes are moved up and out to the opposite or sound eye side, the compensatory head position is face tilt to opposite sound side, chin is depressed and the head tilt to the same side shoulder. The Beilchowksy head tilt is positive on tilting the head towards the normal or sound side. While most of the cases are congenital in origin, it can also occur in trauma to the orbital floor or blow out fracture of the orbit.

Brown's superior oblique tendon sheath syndrome has to be differentiated at times from the inferior oblique paralytic cases. In this syndrome with the forced duction test, there is restriction of passive elevation. Because of changes in superior oblique sheath or muscle it does not relax and does not allow the same sided Inf. oblique to overact.

In inferior oblique palsy, the ipsilateral superior oblique overacts, whereas this generally does not happen with brown superior oblique tendon sheath syndrome. One has to remember that in both of these, there is limitation of movement up and in (to the opposite side), elevation in adduction.

Fourth Cranial Nerve Paralysis

According to Von Noorden[9] (1986), the etiological factors for 4th nerve paralysis in 270 cass treated by the group were (1) congenital, (2) traumatic (closed head-trauma), (3) idiopathic, and (4) neurological; this includes neoplasm and vascular disorders in order of frequency being diabetes, atherosclerosis and hypertension.

With congenital cases, the deviation is present in early life and compensatory head posture (CHP) is a characteristic findings. The patient may not complain of diplopia (a vertical diplopia) whereas in a recently acquired superior oblique paralysis traumatic or vascular in origin, diplopia is a disturbing symptom along with neck strain and tiling of image.

With right superior oblique paralysis and consquent overaction of the ipsilateral inferior oblique, there is hypertropia more marked in the nasal field of the right eye. Later on contracture of the left-sided contralateral inferior rectus muscle, and thereafter weakness or paresis of the left superior rectus results in a CHP. This, however, is seen only in congenital paralytic cases. To differentiate between a superior oblique paralysis (right eye) and superior rectus palsy of the fellow eye (left eye), the head tilt test of Bielchowsky is helpful.

With right superior oblique (RSO) paralysis, the head is tilted to left shoulder, the chin is depressed and the face is turned slightly to left side. With the sound left eye taking up fixation, there is marked hypertropia of the right eye in the primary position. This hypertropia increases when the head is tilted to right shoulder (paralysed side). And when the head is tilted to the sound side (left), the hypertropia gets minimum. On the other hand when the paretic eye (right eye in the case) takes up fixation, there is minimal amount of hypertropia in the paralysed eye (right eye in this case) and the sound left eye is hypotropic due to overaction mainly of the left inferior rectus.

Direct trochlear trauma (trauma to the pulley of superior oblique) as well as a complication of frontal sinus surgery is more common. Occasionally, with closed head-trauma, as in automobile accident, bilateral superior oblique palsy is described.

The patient with congenital or early onset superior oblique palsy is more likely to demonstrate an overacting inferior oblique with a greater deviation in the up position. This is also true of the late onset decompensated patients. Traumatic cases are more likely to demonstrate an overaction of the yoke inferior rectus with a greater deviation in the down position.

Sixth Cranial Nerve Palsy

With sixth cranial nerve paralysis the eye presents the look of a convergent squint (esotropia) but on ocular muscle movement the paralysed eye does not move laterally beyond the mid position as the lateral rectus fails to abduct the eye. The ipsilateral antagonist (the medial rectus) acts unopposed and this may cause esotropia in the primary straight ahead position. The face is turned to the side of paralysed muscle. Etiologically, 6th nerve palsy (lateral rectus paralysis) may be congenital or acquired. A number of congenital cases are bilateral and involve lateral rectus paralysis in both the eyes.

Double Elevator Paralysis

It is a common cause of hyperdeviation. Ocular movements demonstrate a paresis of superior rectus and inferior oblique in the same eye. This may be associated with ptosis when the patient fixes with nonparetic sound eye, the paretic eye will take a hypotropic position and the upper lid may show slight ptosis. On the other hand, fixation with the paralysed will cause hypertropia of the sound eye and ptosis in the paralysed eye may disappear. Conjugate ocular movements are normal in other positions of gaze. The chin is usually elevated.

Etiologically, almost all these cases are congenital in origin though a few cases of acquired paralysis in adult life have also been reported (details in Chapter 13).

In blowout fracture of the orbital floor (see Chapter 15 for details) there may be inability to elevate the eye because of mechanical restriction involving the inferior aspect of the eyeball. But in such cases a forced duction test is positive and this helps to differentiate the two clinical conditions. The treatment is surgical, but when the patient has binocular vision in the primary straight ahead position and has no diplopia except when he attempts to look up and does not show a backward head tilt, surgery is not indicated. Such cases are better left untreated.

Occasionally in such cases an overaction of the superior rectus and inferior oblique of the sound eye is the cause of diplopia and annoyance and needs surgical operation generally myectomy, or recession of the contralateral inferior oblique.

Double depressor paralysis: This involving paralysis of the inferior rectus and superior oblique in one eye, is rare and is mostly congenital in origin. With the sound eye fixing, the paralysed eye is hypertropic in primary position. When fixing with the paretic or affected eye, the sound or non-paretic eye is hypotropic in primary position.

Treatment of Paralytic Squint

The guiding principle in treatment of paralytic squint cases is the presence of diplopia in the primary straight ahead position. In normal use, the eyes generally do not move more than 10° to 15° from this primary position and hence the movement of the eyes in this range should be diplopia-free. Diplopia in extreme position of lateral or vertical gaze is normally easily tolerated or discarded.

Further the inability to maintain binocular single vision without a conspicuous head posture or facial tilt is cosmetically distressing. And thus the aim of treatment is to have a diplopia-free primary position of the eye as also not to allow a compensatory head posture developing. And for these surgery is usually required.

Prisms have been used for relief of diplopia when the deviation is small (less than 10 Δ). But they cannot be used for long periods as also for larger deviation. Further, it is difficult to say that prisms are effective in preventing contractures of the antagonist of a paretic muscle. And thus corrective surgery should be undertaken before contracture has time to develop. Generally, in recent cases of paralysis, a period of six months is allowed for spontaneous recovery along with and after detailed diagnostic examination. In between the patient is frequently examined, symptoms recorded and a record of diplopia field maintained. For visual comfort unilateral occlusion is generally suggested or is preferred.

REFERENCES

1. Boeder P.: Cooperative action of extraocular muscles. *Br. J. Ophthalmol.*, 46: 397, 1967.
2. Burian H. M.: Roman P. J. and Sullivan M. S.: Absence of spontaneous head tilt in superior oblique muscle palsy. *Am. J. Ophthalmol.*, 79: 972, 1975.
3. Chavasse F. B.: In *Worth's Squint or Binocular Reflexes and the Treatment of Strabismus,* 7th edn. London, Bailliere, Tindall & Cox, 1939.
4. Duke Elder, S: *Text Book of Ophthalmology*, Vol. 4. London, Henry Kimpton, 1949.

5. Hardesty H. M.: Diagnosis of paretic vertical rotators. *Am. J. Ophthalmol.*, 56: 811, 1963.
6. Helveston, E. M.: A new two-step method for the diagnosis of isolated cyclovertical muscle palsies. *Am. J. Ophthalmol.*, 64: 914, 1967.
7. Khawam E., Scott A. and Jampolsky A.: Acquired superior oblique palsy: Diagnosis and management. *Arch. Ophthalmol.*, 77 : 761, 1967.
8. Lyle K. and Jackson's: *Practical Orthoptics in the Treatment of Squint*, Rev. 5th edn, Lyle T. K. and Wyber K.G. (eds). London, H. K. Lewis & Co., 1967.
9. Noorden G. K. Von, Murray E. and Wong S. Y.: Superior oblique paralysis—review of 270 cases. *Arch. Ophthalmol.*, 104: 1771, 1986.
10. Parks M. M.: Isolated cyclovertical muscle palsy. *Arch. Ophthalmol.*, 60: 1023, 1958.
11. Rucker C. W.: The causes of paralysis of the third, fourth and sixth cranial nerves. *Am. J. Ophthalmol.*, 61: 1293, 1966.
12. Rush J. A. and Younge B. R.: Paralysis of cranial nerves III, IV and VI: Causes and prognosis in 1,000 cases. *Arch. Ophthalmol.*, 99: 76, 1981.
13. Scott. W. E. and Nank-im S. J.: Isolated inferior oblique paresis. *Arch. Ophthalmol.*, 95: 1585, 1977.
14. Werner D. B., Savino P. J. and Schatz N.: Benign recurrent 6th nerve palsies in childhood. *Arch. Ophthalmol.*, 101: 607, 1983.
15. Znajda J. P. and Krill A. E.: Congenital medial rectus palsy with simultaneous abduction of the two eyes. *Am. J. Ophthalmol.*, 68: 1050, 1969.

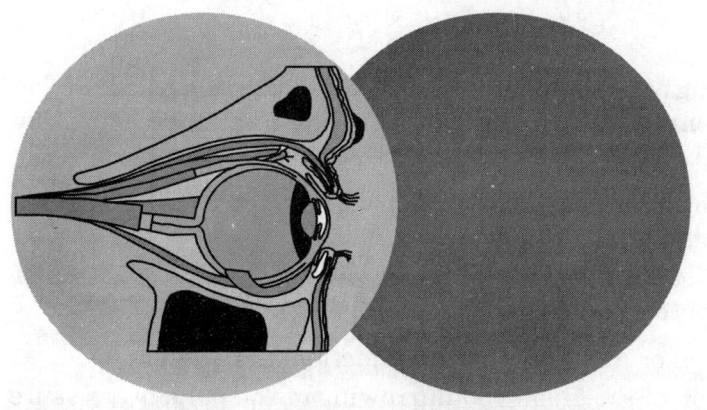

Special Forms of Strabismus
Duane's Retraction Syndrome

On the basis and analysis of clinical findings in 54 cases, Duane in 1905 drew attention to a retraction-syndrome. Since then, this has been mentioned as Duane-retraction syndrome. Still earlier six such cases were described in German literature by Stilling (1887) and Turk (1899). Hence, in the European literature this syndrome is still known as Stilling-Turk-Duane retraction-syndrome.

The classical clinical findings are as follows.

1. Marked limitation of abduction.
2. Slight limitation of adduction.
3. Narrowing of the palpebral fissure on adduction along with retraction of the eyeball.
4. Widening of the palpebral fissure on attempted abduction.
5. Commonly associated elevation or depression in adduction.

Since all such cases do not present similar clinical features, Huber[4,5] suggested the following classification to include most clinical variations in this entity.

DUANE I   • Marked limitation or complete absence of abduction.
            • Normal or only slightly defective adduction.

- Narrowing of the palpebral fissure and retraction on adduction and widening of the palpebral fissure on attempted abduction (Fig. 15.1).

DUANE II
- Limitation or absence of adduction with exotropia of the affected eye, normal or slightly limited abduction
- Narrowing of the palpebral fissure and retraction of the globe on attempted adduction (Fig. 15.2).

DUANE III
- Limitation or absence of both abduction and adduction
- Retraction of the globe and narrowing of the palpebral fissure on attempted adduction.

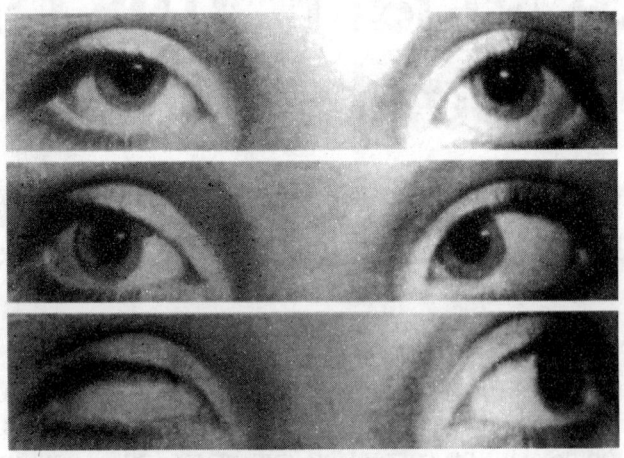

Fig. 15.1: *Duane's retraction syndrome (type I) showing up shoot in adduction in right eye.*

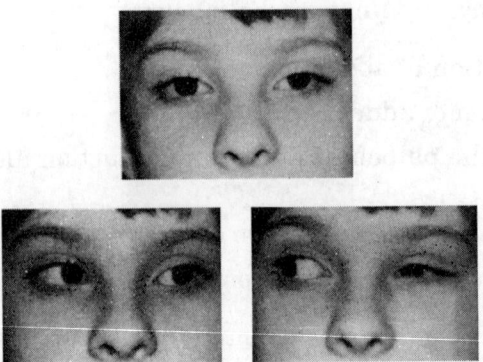

Fig. 15.2: *Duane's retraction syndrome (type II). A child of twelve years age — upper figure slight exotropia right eye, lower left figure shows limited abduction left, lower right figure shows limited adduction of left eye and narrowing of palpebral fissure.*

Duane Type I

It is by far the commonest variety of the syndrome.

In the classical form: An internal squint or esotropia may be present when the eyes are in the primary position. And some would adopt a head-posture to maintain binocular single vision. The frequently associated upshoot and or downshoot of the adducted eye at times causes a cosmetic problem.

At times, other ocular lesions and systemic congenital malformations may be associated with these cases of Duane's retraction syndrome.

Etiology

Things are not as clear, since several factors may be involved in the retraction syndrome, and it is doubtful that a single mechanism is responsible for all such cases.

Anatomical changes involving horizontal rectus muscles have been mentioned. Thus Turk (1899) believed that fixation of the globe by a nonelastic lateral rectus muscle was the cause of retraction on adduction. Many have found during surgery a fibrotic nonelastic lateral rectus muscle or restricting fibrous bands beneath the muscle insertion.

Heuck found a relatively posterior insertion of the medial rectus muscle which he thought to be the cause of retraction of the globe on adduction.

The abnormal vertical eye movements of upshoot or downshoot that frequently occur with adduction have been blamed as due to overaction of the oblique muscles.

Electromyographic studies indicate that an innervational mechanism is more important etiologically than the anatomical anomalies. Thus Breinen[2] described the paradoxic electrical behaviour of the lateral rectus muscle in such patients, that is, absence of electrical activity in this muscle on abduction and active electrical potential on adduction.

Treatment

Surgery is indicated only when:

1. There is a significant deviation in the primary position which is cosmetically disturbing; this deviation is generally esotropia (but may be exotropia in Duane II cases), and
2. binocular single vision cannot be maintained without a significant anomalous head-tilt and which is also not cosmetically desirable.

However, with a small degree of deviation and a feasible binocular single vision with a slight head-turn, one would not like to operate on such cases as results have not been convincing.

When esotropia is present, a 5 mm recession of the ipsilateral medial rectus is undertaken. This, however, does not improve motility in abduction but is successful in minimising head-turn.

On the operation table under general anaesthesia, a forced duction-test is invaluable in deciding whether retraction is caused by a fibrotic lateral rectus muscle or by synergistic innervation of both horizontal muscles.

When there is resistance on passive adduction, the lateral rectus muscle is more likely fibrotic.

On the other hand, when there is no resistance to passive adduction, paradoxic innervation must be considered and resection of the lateral rectus muscle is not indicated. Otherwise it may cause increased retraction in adduction.

Duane II and III

In Duane II cases with exotropia in the primary position, recession of the lateral rectus muscle of the involved eye may be considered.

In Duane III cases with limitation of abduction and abduction surgery may not be rewarding.

Thus, it would appear that in these cases no rigid rule could be laid down for the surgical treatment as also the procedure for surgical treatment. An individualised approach taking into account the horizontal and vertical deviation is the need and necessity.

Superior Oblique Tendon Sheath (Brown's) Syndrome

The clinical features of Brown's syndrome (Figs. 15.3 and 15.4) are as follows. The patient has straight eyes or slight hypotropia in the primary position.

1. In adduction, elevation is absent or not feasible, but
2. Normal or near normal elevation in primary position and also in abduction.
3. Positive forced duction test (restriction of passive elevation).
4. Divergence in upward gaze (V-pattern).
5. Less commonly:
   a. Frequent depression of the eye in adduction,
   b. occasional overaction of the ipslateral superior oblique, and
   c. occasional widening of the palpebral fissure on adduction.

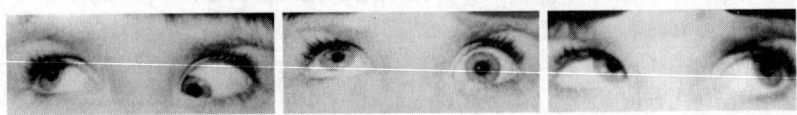

Fig. 15.3:   *Brown's syndrome: In this case the left sided figure shows inability to elevate the left eye in adduction. This is also present in the primary position (central figure) while the elevation is normal in abduction (right figure).*

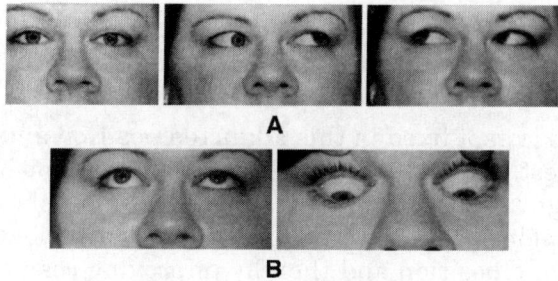

Fig. 15.4: **A.** *Left sided figure shows primary position with normal alignment. Central figure shows elevation right eye limited in adduction on up and left gaze. Right figure shows normal up and right movement.*
B. *Left figure shows normal up gaze and right figure shows normal down gaze.*

The clinical features thus, very much resemble paralysis of inferior oblique muscle of the same side, the direction of the head-tilt being on the same side and the chin is raised. Diplopia is usually elicited when the involved eye is adducted. It is avoided in the primary position by anomalous head position. That the contralateral superior rectus instead of showing overaction shows a normal action and the positive forced duction test of superior oblique clearly differentiates inferior oblique palsy from the Brown's syndrome.

Etiology

According to Brown, the fault lies with the sheath of the superior oblique muscle which according to him is congenitally short. Occasionally, there may be a series of fibrous band between the tendon and sheath. After the sheath has been dissected, normalization of the forced duction test indicates that the fault is primarily in the sheath. A few cases have been described wherein the clinical features of Brown's syndrome have appeared following tucking of superior oblique tendon indicating further that the fault lies with the superior oblique tendon.

Treatment

When the involved eye is hypotropic in the primary position or where there is a significant abnormal head posture, surgery may be attempted to restore binocular single vision in primary position.

Otherwise in those, where binocular vision is normal and comfortable in primary position and there is not much cosmetic problem of abnormal head posture, it is better to leave these cases as such.

To dissect and strip off the sheath while leaving the tendon of superior oblique intact, or a complete tenectomy[4] of the superior oblique are surgical procedures with their favourites and opposing surgeons.

Strabismus Fixus

It is a rare clinical condition in which one (or sometimes both eyes) eye is always in a position of extreme adduction.

The involved eye is as if fixed in this adducted position and cannot be moved. A forced duction test will confirm that the eyeball cannot be moved laterally (abducted). Thought to be caused by congenital fibrosis of medial rectus, treatment is surgical in such cases. The medial rectus muscle is recessed bringing the eyeball to midline position and thereby improving cosmetic and functional improvement.

A divergent type of strabismus fixus is still a rarity.

Cyclic Heterotropia or Alternate Day Esotropia[13]

It is a fascinating form of esotropia seen in a young child. It follows a 48 hours of rhythm, that is, a 24 hours period of binocular single vision followed by 24 hours of manifest esotropia. On the day when there is no deviation (esotropia) or straight eye day, no anomaly of binocular single vision can be detected. On the day of esotropia a large angle esotropia will appear, and sensory anomalies may be found. Occasionally diplopia may be complained of. This cyclic nature of squint may last for several years and thereafter, esotropia may become constant. The mechanism of the cyclic heterophoria is obscure. In some cases a strong family history of strabismus may be obtained. So far treatment is concerned, such cases have to be kept under observation for a number of years for the nature to help. In those with marked strabismus on squint day, conventional surgery for esotropia may be done taking care to be on the safe side that is under correction.

Thyroid Myopathy[6, 7]

Two distinct clinical conditions have to be recognised, viz.

(1) Grave's disease or goitre seen generally in young women with proptosis, lid-retraction, lid-lag, tremor and a variety of ocular findings; and the (2) Second one known by a variety of names as exophthalmic ophthalmoplegia, endocrine exophthalmos, dysthyroid eye disease and exophthalmic goitre, is a clinical condition affecting middle aged individuals.

A few of these patients have the history of thyroidectomy a few years back and some of them have been treated in the past for transient episodes of hyperthyroidism. But a number of them start spontaneously with periorbital transient oedema and limitations of elevation of one or both eyes. Evidence of hypothyroidism or lack of adequate thyroid function on detailed clinical examination and laboratory tests may be found in a few others.

Detailed clinical evaluation of such cases may reveal exophthalmos and limitation of ocular motility in several or all directions caused by marked swelling and congestion of retrobulbar orbital contents. But in classical cases, as mentioned above, the first symptom to draw attention is frequent and transient periorbital oedema (subsiding in between) and limitation of elevation of one eye.

Treatment

In those with hyperthyroidism, medical treatment is the first line of treatment with antithyroid drugs. In those with marked edema and increasing exophthalmos, high doses of corticosteroids have been found useful. Once the deviation has stabilised, surgery becomes the treatment of choice. A large recession of the inferior rectus muscles is indicated when elevation is limited. But this may be debatable. Adjustable sutures may be used to correct for overcorrection or undercorrections.

For limitation of abduction, a large recession of medial rectus may be necessary.

Many patients affected with this disease, have to bear with vertical diplopia for many months specially those in whom undue swelling of muscle (inferior rectus) and tightness of tissues does not allow recession to be carried out.

Fracture of the Orbital Floor (Blow out Fracture)

A blunt injury to the eye and consequent impaction of the globe backwards causes increased orbital pressure and the orbit tends to give way at its weakest point—the orbital floor.[14] Orbital contents such as fat, fascia, the inferior rectus muscle and inferior oblique muscle or sometimes the entire globe may prolapse in the maxillary-antrum and part of these (tissue) may get incarcerated into the fracture track.

Occasionally a blowout fracture of the medial wall opening into the ethmoid sinus may be produced causing emphysema of the retro bulbar area.

Proptosis commonly occurs during the immediate posttraumatic phase along with marked swelling and ecchymosis of the lids and periorbital tissue.

On examination there is marked limitation of eye movements, particularly elevation and depression. Once the eyeball can be opened, diplopia is complained of.

Careful ophthalmic examination is necessary in all such cases of orbital injuries. X-ray examination supplemented by a CT scan and MRI may be necessary to demonstrate a crack or a fracture in the bony structure of the orbital floor.

Early surgery is not indicated in all such cases of orbital injuries even though X-rays or CT scan may indicate crack-fracture in orbital floor. This is more so in those who do not complain of diplopia. Conservative medical treatment should be carried out. This reduces edema and swelling of periorbital tissues as also helps in improving ocular motility.

However, once it is found that there is no significant improvement of ocular motility and the radiographic findings are positive for a fracture and forcedduction test indicates incarceration of orbital tissue, surgery should not be delayed. This is all the more indicative when there is exophthalmos. An ENT surgeon may have to be associated in surgery to open the maxillary antrum and help in elevating the tissues of the orbital floor that have drawn into the antrum. Plastic repair of orbital floor has to be done thereafter.

REFERENCES

1. Beck M. and Hickling P.: Treatment of bilateral superior oblique sheath syndrome complicating rheumatoid arthritis. *Br. J. Ophthalmol.* 64: 358, 1980.
2. Breinin G. M.: Electromyography — a tool in ocular and neurological diagnosis II: Muscle palsies. *Arch. Ophthalmol.*, 57: 165, 1957.
3. Costenbadar, E. D. and Albert D. G.: Spontaneous regression of pseudoparalysis of the inferior oblique muscle. *Arch. Ophthalmol.*, 59 : 607, 1958.
4. Duke Elder S.: *Text Book of Ophthalmology*, Vol 4. London, Henry Kimpton, 1949.
5. Duke Elder S.: *System of Ophthalmology*, Vol 3, *Congenital Deformities*. St. Louis, C. V. Mosby Co., 1963.
6. Glaser J.: Grave's ophthalmopathy (editorial). *Arch. Ophthalmol.*, 102: 1448, 1984.
7. Goldstein J. E.: Paresis of superior rectus muscle associated with thyroid dysfunction. *Arch. Ophthalmol.*, 72 : 5, 1964.
8. Grawford J. S., Orton R. and Labow Daily L: Late results of superior oblique muscle tenotomy in true Brown's syndrome. *Am. J. Ophthalmol.*, 89: 824, 1980.
9. Khodadoust A. A. and Noordan G. K. Von: Bilateral vertical retraction syndrome. *Arch. Ophthalmol.*, 78 : 606, 1967.
10. Lyle T. K. and Bridgemam G. J. O.: *Worth and Chavase's Squint: The binocular reflexes and the treatment of strabismus*, 9th edn. London, Bailliere Tindall & Cox, 1959.
11. Mein J.: Alternating inferior oblique palsy. *Br. Orthop. J.*, 21: 116, 1964.
12. Parks M. M.: The weakening surgical procedures for eliminating overaction of the inferior oblique muscle. *Am. J. Ophthalmol.*, 73: 107, 1972.
13. Roper Hall, M. J. and Yapt J. M. S.: Alternate day squint, In *Proc. First International Congress of Orthoptics*, 1968. St. Louis, The C. V. Mosby Co.
14. Smith B. and Regan E. F.: Blowout fracture of the orbit — mechanism and correction of the internal orbital fracture. *Am. J. Ophthalmol.*, 44: 733, 1959.
15. Stanworth A: Ocular myopathies. *Trans Ophthal. Soc., U. K.*, 83: 515, 1953.

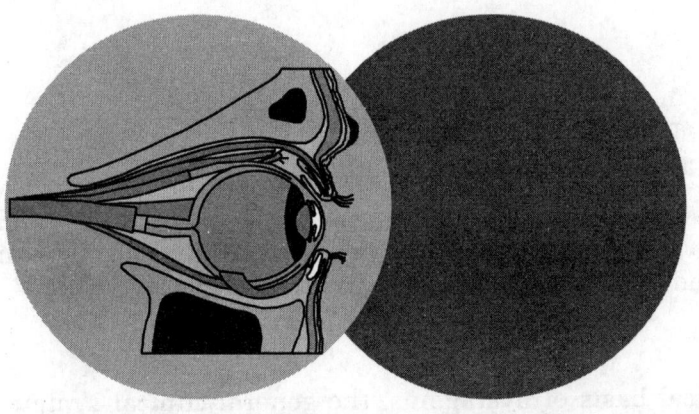

Nystagmus

Nystagmus may be defined as an involuntary, repetitive, rhythmic, coordinated movement or oscillation of the eye usually affecting both eyes. The oscillations may be pendular or jerky in nature.

In the pendular type of nystagmus, both phases of the movement are of equal speed. Such movement or oscillation may occur in any plane depending on the etiology. Thus, it may be horizontal (commonest type), vertical or rotatory.

In the jerky type of nystagmus the movement consists of a slow phase in one direction followed by a quick phase in the opposite direction. The slow phase is the fundamental one, whereas the jerky phase in the opposite direction is compensatory to bring back the eyes to their normal primary position. According to the direction of the quick phase, the nystagmus is labelled as to the left, right, up or down.

Some forms of nystagmus are normal. Thus nystagmus that occurs in response to rotation of an optokinetic drum or rotation of the body in space acts to preserve clear vision. Nystagmus can also be produced experimentally in normal individuals. And this provides evidence of value as to the role of the vestibular apparatus and of the eyes in producing nystagmus.

Etiology and Types

Nystagmus could be broadly divided into the following types depending on the etiological factors.

1. Ocular-nystagmus.
2. Labrynthine and vestibular nystagmus.
3. Nystagmus of central origin.

The ocular type of nystagmus includes amongst others, the voluntary and hysterical nystagmus as also the congenital type. Each group has its own characteristic features and different approach to treatment.

Symptomatology

Whatever be the etiological basis of nystagmus, the general clinical symptomatology is more or less similar. In the congenital type of nystagmus (mostly ocular in origin) symptoms are negligible. The eyes move but to the individual, objects do not appear to move. Visual acuity is usually poor which is basically the cause of nystagmus and not so much its effect. There are, however, cases in which the visual acuity is relatively good despite the oscillations of the eyeball.

On the other hand, in the acquired type of nystagmus symptoms are greatly pronounced. The patient feels giddy, has vertigo and nausea. This happens mostly in nystagmus of labrynthine origin as also in miner's nystagmus.

Diplopia Ocular nystagmus is not characterised by diplopia.

Tilting of head So that the gaze is directed away from the direction where the nystagmus-amplitude is the greatest head is tilted to minimise the apparent movement of objects and blurring of vision.

Head tremor Sometimes accompanies the ocular nystagmus. Ocular nystagmus is usually pendular in type with greater rapidity or extremely slow rate of movement. It may, thus, demonstrate varying amplitude, both great and small.

Nystagmus of central origin is generally absent in the primary position and occurs only on conjugate deviation of the eyes sideways or upwards. It is generally jerky in nature.

Labrynthine nystagmus is usually associated with marked symptoms of giddiness, vertigo and nausea. It is usually jerky in type and seen mostly in sideways.

OCULAR NYSTAGMUS

Ocular nystagmus is due to an embarrassment of or to a defect of central vision, which makes fixation difficult or impossible.

A healthy macula consisting only of cones is not fully developed till the fourth to sixth months of life. A newborn baby is not able to fix the eyes on an object, nor is able to follow a moving object in a steady manner. Thus, a normally developed fovea is the prime necessity for fixation. Consequently, in poor macular fixation resulting from imperfect development or disease (before the age of fixation usually upto six months of neonatal life) ocular nystagmus results.

The various types of ocular nystagmus are as follows.

A. Physiologically Induced Nystagmus

i. *Deviational nystagmus*: When the eyes are deviated to their extreme lateral excursions so that fixation becomes difficult.

ii. *Opto-kinetic nystagmus*: When fixation is confused by a succession of rapidly moving objects traversing the visual field.

iii. *Latent nystagmus*: Occasionally if one eye is covered.

B. Pathological

i. Congenital manifest nystagmus (CMN)
   a. Infantile idiopathic nystagmus
   b. Sensory defect nystagmus due to a variety of obvious or subtle disorders such as congenital-cataract, dense corneal-leucoma, optic disc atrophy, etc.

ii. Nystagmus due to blindness or amaurotic nystagmus.

iii. Nystagmus due to defective central vision seen in albinism, and achromatopsia, etc.

iv. Spasmus nutans.

v. Miner's nystagmus.

Voluntary Nystagmus

Herein, the movements are pendular, horizontal and very rapid. It is a habit learnt. There is always an apparent movement of objects. It is rare for the quivering to be kept up for longer than half a minute owing to giddiness, headache, and fatigue.

Hysterical nystagmus may show all the features of the voluntary type and the pendular oscillations tend to be even quicker.

Physiologically Induced Ocular Nystagmus

Deviational or End-position Nystagmus

An example is the train nystagmus when eyes follow a tree from inside the moving train. As the tree gets out of focus, the eyes roll back to normal position with a jerk to fixate another tree in the scenery after a latent period of a few seconds. It occurs more readily if there is a paresis of an extraocular muscle.

The nystagmus in such circumstances tends to be irregular rather than being pendular.

Opto-kinetic Nystagmus

This is another example of a deviational nystagmus provoked by visual stimuli under controlled conditions. The patient is seated on a chair in front of a revolving drum with black and white stripes on its outer surface. To elicit the nystagmus, three conditions are necessary — a normal functioning fovea, attention on the part of the patient and presence of contours in the panorma. Hence, if the fovea is diseased or not fully developed or the moving object does not attract attention, optokinetic nystagmus is not elicited.

The occurrence of optokinetic nystagmus depends primarily on the fixation and refixation reflexes as it is mediated by the cortical centres independently of the subcortical mechanism. Interest and attention on the moving objects are required and sufficient activity in the afferent sensory path to convey the impression, is a must. Lesions affecting the higher visual cortex and their associational tract or the motor tract to the oculomotor muscles will abolish the response.

In an infant suspected of blindness, failure to elicit optokinetic nystagmus is a confirmation of blindness unless the infant is mentally deficient.

Latent (Manifest Latent) Nystagmus

In the condition of latent nystagmus, the nystagmus is not ordinarily present when both eyes are open. It is elicited by covering either of the eyes. There is no obvious pathological condition of the media, fundi or visual tract.

The typical features of the latent nystagmus are as follows.

1. When both eyes are open and the visual axes are directed straight forward, the eyes are steady. There is slight jerking nystagmus on lateral movements of the eyes.
2. On covering one or the other eye, bilateral nystagmus is evoked.
3. The nystagmus is of horizontal and jerking type with the rapid phase towards the side of the uncovered eye or fixing eye. Occlusion of the right eye causes a strong jerking nystagmus with its quick phase to the left.
4. The visual acuity is decreased as soon as the nystagmus occurs. When there is no nystagmus, the visual acuity is better but as soon as one eye is occluded the visual acuity of the other eye also goes down.
5. The nystagmus is less pronounced and the visual acuity improved if the head is turned so that the eye under observation is adducted.
6. The nystagmus is present from infancy and may be associated with squint.
7. When the weaker eye (the eye with poor visual acuity) is occluded, the nystagmus is fine. On the other hand when the stronger eye is occluded, the nystagmus is coarse. Sometimes, if one eye has very poor vision, on covering the better eye instead of nystagmus a conjugate deviation of both eyes occurs towards the side of the closed eye—latent deviation of Kestenbaum (1921).

PATHOLOGICAL NYSTAGMUS

Nystagmus in infancy may be present at birth, but frequently appears in the first six months of life. It can be classified as congenital manifest nystagmus

(CMN), sensory defect nystagmus and nystagmus associated with neurological disease.

Congenital manifest nystagmus (CMN) or also called *Infantile idiopathic nystagmus:* A normal child presenting with typical CMN-reduced visual acuity (0.3 or better) and no other neurological or ocular defect could be diagnosed as congenital manifest nystagmus (CMN) without further investigation. Such a nystagmus is generally pendular and horizontal and shows no change (on occluding one eye). It is infrequently associated with infantile esotropia. The binocular visual acuity is same as the monocular visual acuity. And this is generally less than normal. Visual acuity at near-fixation distance often is dramatically better than at distance fixation. Hence, one should always check the visual acuity both at distance and at near.

Some patients with congenital manifest nystagmus are able to decrease the amplitude or frequency of the nystagmus by superimposed convergence, the phenomenon being known as dampening or blockage (nystagmus blockage syndrome). The purpose of such dampening is to improve visual acuity.

Another dampening strategy used by patients with nystagmus (CMN) is version innervation. Maintaining the eyes in a peripheral gaze position by sustained innervation of yoke muscles involved in lateral, vertical or oblique gaze causes dampening of nystagmus innervation. The result is that the child would assume a significant anomalous headposture in an effort to gain optimal visual acuity and with least amplitude of nystagmic movement. Depending on the preferred eyeposition (null-point or neutral zone, when the nystagmus is least evident) the head may be turned to either side, tilted towards one shoulder or the chin may be elevated or depressed. But this anomalous head-posture may not always be in one direction. The child should, therefore, be observed for several minutes to check for periodic alternating nystagmus (PAN) where the null-zone shifts with tilt.

Sensory defect nystagmus: Also called secondary nystagmus, it is the most common form of congenital nystagmus, and is secondary to a variety of obvious or subtle disorders such as congenital cataract, corneal leucoma, optic atrophy and albinism, etc.

Nystagmus in them results from inadequate image-formation on the fovea as a result of anterior-visual-pathway disease. This (inadequate image formation) causes a disturbance of the feedback from the fovea and that interferes with ocular-motor control of the fixation mechanism.

Clinically such a nystagmus is bilateral, horizontal and often pendular in type in which the eyes oscillate with equal velocity in both directions.

Nystagmus may develop in a child months after the onset of congenital cataract who previously had no nystagmus or it may disappear after cataract surgery followed by contact lens correction. Hence, there may not be a causal relationship in all such cases.

Nystagmus due to blindness Nystagmus either pendular or jerky in type may occur in those who have been blind for a long time. It may be constant or it may occur only when the attention is aroused. In an infant born blind, the movement is irregular, variable and of large excursion.

Nystagmus due to defective central vision (amblyopic- nystagmus) which precludes the normal development of the fixation reflex is generally noticed during the first few months of life when the child begins to make efforts to fix. If amblyopia develops after fixation has been acquired, nystagmus does not usually appear. It is bilateral amblyopia which causes nystagmus to develop. In the unilateral amblyopia, on the other hand, strabismus is the result.

Common causes are albinism, albinoidism (hypopigmentation), achromatopsia, congenital or infantile ocular anomalies in the media or retina which make fixation difficult or impossible in early life. Such an amblyopic nystagmus varies considerably in the direction, rapidity and extent of movement. It may be fine ryhthmic movement of the eyes or so coarse and rapid that examination of the fundus may be impossible.

Spasmus nutans In this condition nystagmus is associated with head nodding movement commencing usually at the age of 6 or 7 months of neonatal life and persisting for not more than a year or so. The nystagmus is pendular in type and of rapid frequency. It may be horizontal, vertical or rotatory. The head-nodding may appear earlier than the nystagmus and the head movement may be vertical, rotatory or horizontal. And this occurs in short series alternating with periods of rest.

Miner's nystagmus Coal miners who had to work for prolonged period of time in the ill-ventitlated and poorly illuminated coal mines did suffer from nystagmus which has been called miner's nystagmus. The essential factor in its production is dim-illumination in association with a disturbance of the vertibular apparatus as a result of the couched attitude of the miner which necessitates a constant upward gaze and mental fatigue. Lack of proper ventilation and inhalation of poisonous gases down in the mines added to the etiology.

The nystagmus is horizontal in nature and typically present in the upper field of gaze it may also be oblique in type. Mental symptoms are generally associated alongwith head-retraction, blepharospasm, dizziness, headache and vertigo, etc.

Fortunately, with improved illumination and working conditions in the mines, such a nystagmus is generally not seen these days.

Management of Nystagmus

The treatment of these various types of ocular nystagmus depends essentially on the cause, and the management options available are both nonsurgical and surgical.

Decreased foveation time and image movement are the possible factors responsible for reduced vision and amblyopia. In nystagmus, reducing eye oscillation is, thus, suggested to increase foveation time and reduce movement of image on the retina, thereby bringing about improvement of vision.

Most patients with congenital nystagmus try to improve their visual performance by holding the object of regard very close to the eyes. This induces convergence which dampens the amplitude and frequency of nystagmus. Others adopt an abnormal head-posture with the eyes directed into an eccentric gaze position. This also tends to dampen the nystagmus and improve visual acuity. The commonest posture is a face turn to one side, the less common being tilt of the head or elevating or depressing the chin.

The visual acuity must be measured with and without a head-posture, if present. Following are some of the non-surgical management procedures.

1. All cases require a good cycloplegic refraction as many patients are astigmatic and anisometropic. A prescription of appropriate glasses does sometimes help in stabilising the nystagmus.

Concave (minus) lenses have been used to stimulate accommodation and secondarily covergence which in turn would and could improve ocular stability.

2. Prism: Base out prisms may be used to stimulate convergence and thereby to stabilise the eyes. These prisms may be prescribed with the base towards the head-turn to allow eccentric ocular position and straight head. With a head turn to the left, the neutral zone is dextro-version. Herein, a prism with base-in before the right eye and base out before the left eye will correct the head tilt.

However, since large dioptre prisms which may have to be used in such cases are heavy, they are cosmetically not appreciated. They are probably best used diagnostically to decide if surgery would help or to deal with small residual head-turn after surgery.

3. Drugs and botulinum toxin injection into extraocular muscles have also been tried.

Surgical Treatment

Surgery in nystagmus is usually performed to correct head-posture and to improve vision by decreasing the amplitude or frequency of nystagmus.

In 1953, Kestenbaum (quoted by Noorden[10]) recommended surgical shifting of the eyes by identical amount of recession and resection in the direction of the rapid phase of nystagmus away from the nullpoint. Thus, for a head-turn to the left Kestenbaum first operated in the right eye-recession of the right lateral rectus and resection of the right medial rectus. In a second operation he took the left eye recession of the left medial rectus and resection of the left lateral rectus. He advocated performing an equal amount of surgery (5 mm) on all the four muscles.

Anderson[2] in the same year (1953) recessed the yoke muscle in each eye. Thus for a head turn to the left he recessed the right lateral rectus and left medial rectus. Parks (1973)[11] advocated his modification of the Kestenbaum procedure, calling it 5-6-7-8 procedure.

With recession of one medial rectus 5 mm and one (LE) lateral rectus 7 mm with resection of the other medial rectus 6 mm and recession of other lateral rectus 8 mm.

If a squint is present, it is possible to add algebrically the amount of surgery required remembering to do the required surgery on the fixing eye as that determines the head turn.

Another surgical procedure is symmetrical recession of the four horizontal rectus muscles. By retroplacement of horizontal rectus muscle insertions behind the equator and posterior to the tangential plane, their leverage is decreased and a given amount of muscle innvervation will have less rotational effect on the globe. In cases of nystagmus, this would cause a decrease in amplitude (Noordan[10]).

It is advocated that for anomalous head posture caused by manifest nystagmus, surgery should be delayed till the child is at least four years old. Repeated visits and evaluation are advisable to establish the direction, constancy and degree of anomalous head-posture which may not be easily obtainable in younger children.

REFERENCES

1. Abardiv R.V. and Whittle J.: Surgery and compensatory head posture in congenital nystagmus — a longitudinal study. *Arch Ophthal.*, 110, 632-5: 1992.
2. Anderson J.R.: Causes and treatment of Congenital nystagmus. *Br. J. Ophthalmol.*, 37 : 267, 1953.
3. Duke-Elder W.: *Textbook of Ophthalmology*, Vol. IV, London, Henry Kimpton, 1949.
4. Harcourt B: Faden operation (postfixation sutures). *Eye*, Vol. 2, part I, 36-40 (1988).
5. Huban Atilla, Necile Akran, Yusuf Isikcelik: Surgical treatment in nystagmus. *Eye*, 13, (pt I): 11-15, 1999.
6. John S. Stahl, Lea Averbuch-Heller, R. John Leigh. Acquired nystagmus. *Arch Ophthalmol,* 118, 544, 2000.
7. Lee J.P.: Surgical management of nystagmus, *Eye*, 2 (Pt I): 44-7, 1988.
8. Lyle and Jacksons: *Practical Orthoptics in the Treatment of Squint*, 5th edn. London, H.K. Lewis, 1967.
9. Noorden G.K. Von: Binocular vision and ocular mobility, 4th edn. St. Louis, C.V. Mosby Co., 1990.
10. Noorden G.K. Von, Springer D.T.: Large rectus muscle recessions for the treatment of congenital nystagmus. *Arch Ophthal*, 109: 221-4, 1991.
11. Parks M. M.: Congenital nystagmus surgery. *Am Orthopt J.*, 23: 35, 1973.

Index

A & V pattern/syndrome   164
   clinical picture   169
   etiology   166-167
   indication for surgery   171
   treatment   169-170
Abnormal retinal correspondence   73-76,
     80
Acommodation–convergence
     anomalies   39
   ratio
     high   143
     normal   46
Adapatation to strabismus   67
After-image   78
Amblyopia
   classification & terminology   80
   definition   80
   treatment-oclusion   87
   miotics-penalisation   89
   red filter   88
Anatomy of extraocular muscle   1
Angle of deviation   59
   alpha   59
   gamma   59
   kappa   59
   clinical significance   64
   examination on synoptophore   62

Bagolini striated lens test   79
Binocular vision   26

Convergence
   anomalies   41-43
   excess   45
   insufficiency   44
   reflex   43

Duane's retraction syndrome   203-205
Diplopia-confusion   67-68

Esotropia   142-154
   clinical types   142-143
   treatment
     medical   153
     surgical   108-109
Exotropia   155
   clinical types   156

intermittent   161
   treatment   160
Extraocular muscle
   anatomy   1-14
   movement
     uniocular   12
     binocular   12
   nerve supply   11

Functional amblyopia in
     alternative squint   80
   eccentric fixation   88
   occlusion-therapy   87
   CAM   90

Grave's disease   208

Head posture in AV pattern
   in paralytic squint   186
   in nystagmus   212
Head - tilt   212, 186
Hess screen test   191-193
Heterophoria
   symptoms in   130
   etiology of   131

Hirschberg-test   59-60
Homonymous diplopia   69-70
Horopter   29

Illiterate E chart in estimation of visual
     acuity of children   54
Incomitant strabismus   182
Infantile strabismus   146
Inferior oblique muscle   6
   action of   19
   overaction of   122
   paralysis of   199
Inferior rectus muscle   2
   action of   12
Insufficiency of convergence-othoptics in
     treatment of   44-45

Kestenbaum-Anderson procedure   217

Latent and manifest-latent congenital
     nystamus   214

Ligaments of lockwood   10

Metre angle   41
Maddox wing   133
   rod   134
Major amblyoscope measurement
      with   101
Manifest congenital nystagums   250
Manifest strabismus   215
Medial rectus muscle   3
      action of   12
      paralysis   198
      recession   120

Microtropia   150
Miotics
   action of   103
   effect of on acommodative-convergence/
      accommodation ratio   103
   indications for   103
   in treatment of amblyopia   104

Movement, eye   15-16
   cardinal   19

Near vision complex   39
   accommodation in   40

Nerve III paralysis   197
Nerve IV paralysis   199
Nerve VI paralysis   200

Non-accommodative esotropia   143, 146,
      148
Non-surgical treatment, principles of
   optical   95
   bifocals   96
   prims in   97
   spectacles   95
   orthoptics in   100

Pharmacological
   atropine   90
   botulinum injection   103
   miotics in   103

Nystagmus
   congenital   255
   characteristic of   211
   latent   213
   manifest-latent   214
   medical treatment of   216
   surgical treatment of   217

Nystagmus blockage syndome   215

Nystagmus dampening syndrome   215-
      217

Oblique muscles   5-6
   action of   12-19
   overaction of inferior oblique   122
Occlusion
   direct   97-98, 87-88
   inverse   88, 99
   in treatment of amblyopia   98
Ocular movements   15-25
Operation
   amount of   119-120
Optokinetic nystagms   213
Orbital floor, fractures of   180
Orthoptics
   cam treatment in   90-91, 99
   drugs   103
   occlusion in   87-88
   penalisation in
   pleoptics in   89
   prisms in   97
   red filter in   98
   for exophoria   139

Recession
   of rectus muscle   113
Rectus muscles
   action of   12
   insertion of   2-4
   measurement of   112-113
   strengthening of   116
   weakening of   113
Red filter treatment of amblyopia   88
Refraction   144
   in concomitant strabisms   144
   accommodative convergence/
      accomodation ratio Ac/A   143
Retinal correspondence anomalies   73
Retraction syndrome (Duane's)
   clinical findings and diagnosis of   204,
      205, 206
   etiology of   205
Rod maddox   134

Secondary overaction of inferior oblique
      muscle   122
Single binocular vision, Panum's area
      of   29, 30, 31
Small angle esotropia/exotropia   150
Strabismus
   A - V pattern   164-166
   etiology of   165-173
   concomitant infantile   108, 146
   paralytic   182, 202

Strengthening operation   116, 117, 118
Striated glass test of Bagolini   79
Superior oblique muscle tendon sheath
      syndrome (Brown)   206, 207
Superior rectus muscle
  action of   3
  paralysis of   198
  recession of   131
Suppession   69-70
  alternating   70-72
  clinical features of   70, 71, 72
Surgical techniques   113-124
Sutures
  adjustable sutures   113-114
  posterior fixation (Faden
      operation)   115-116

Tangent-scale   138
Tendon

of inferior oblique   6
of rectus muscle   1
of superior oblique   5, 112
Tenon's capsule   7-8
Torticollis   196

Uncrossed diplopia   68, 71

V - esotropia   115
V - exotropia   108-111
Vertical rectus muscles, action of   12-13
Visual acuity   52-53
Visual axis teminology   59

Weakening operation   113-116
Worth 4 dot. test   62, 63
Zinn annulus of   2